Cultural Competency Skills for Psychologists, Psychotherapists, and Counselling Professionals

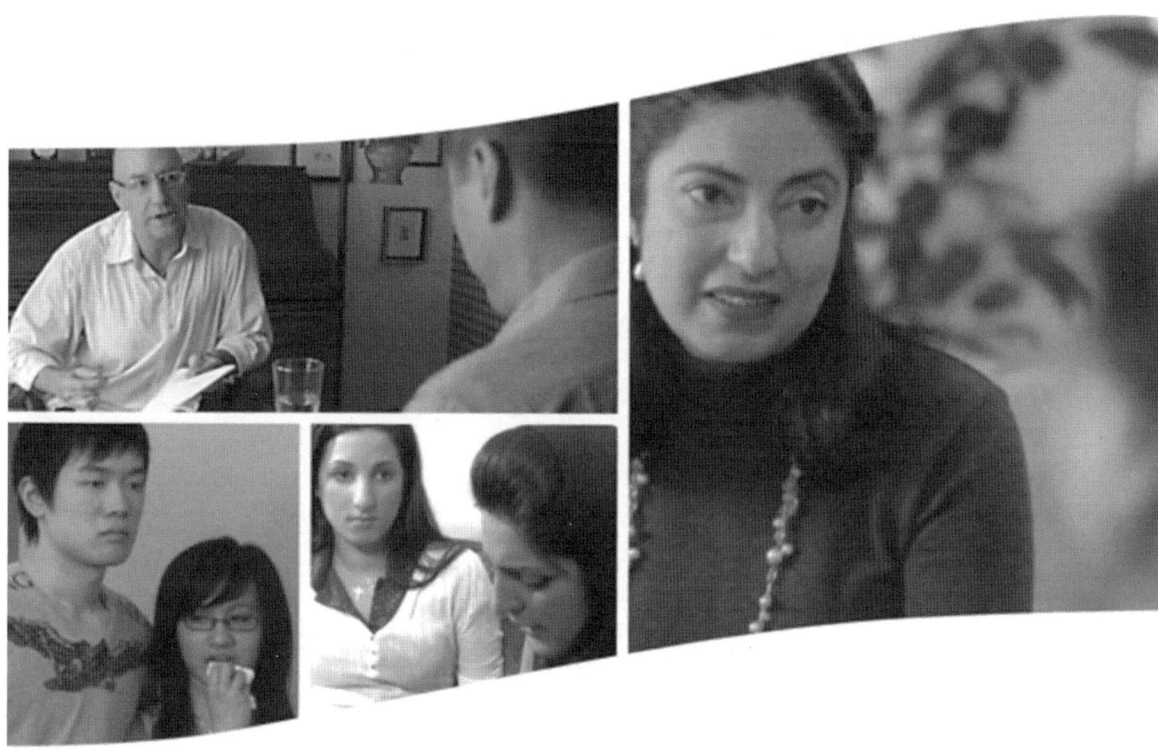

Cultural Competency Skills for Psychologists, Psychotherapists, and Counselling Professionals

A WORKBOOK FOR CARING ACROSS CULTURES

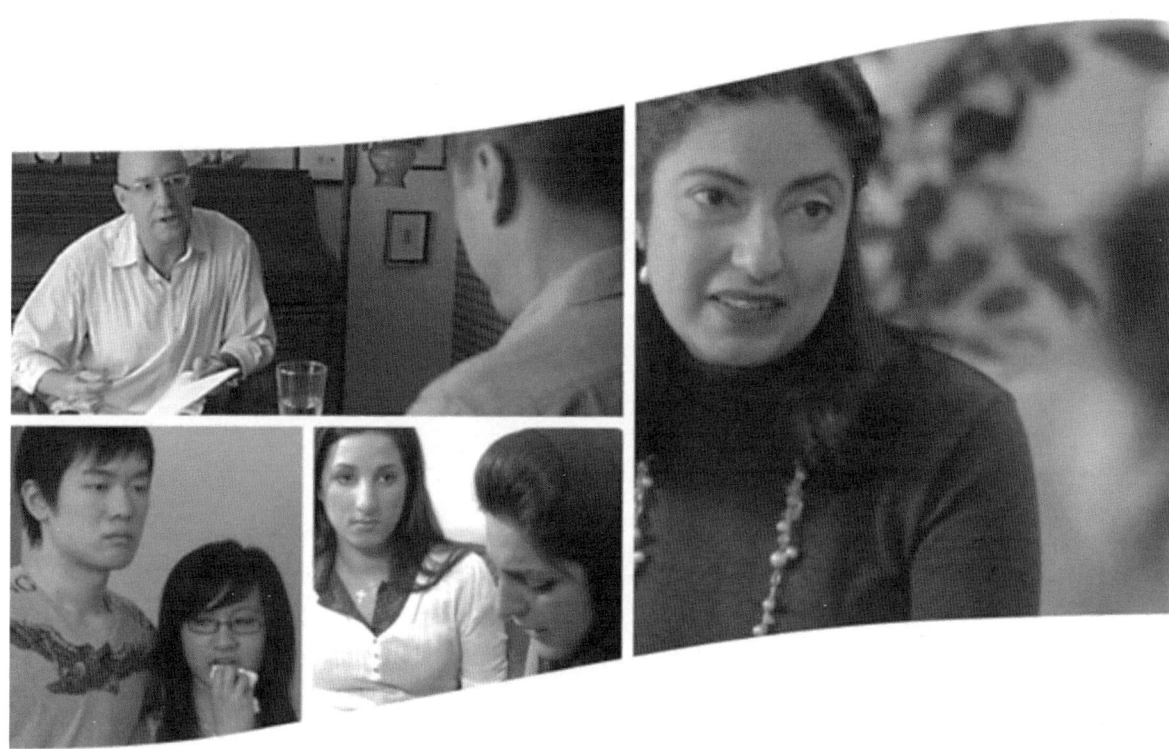

EARLE WAUGH

OLGA SZAFRAN

JEAN A. C. TRISCOTT

ROGER PARENT

Psychology Team: Roger Gervais, Wes Penner, Carolyn Triscott, Sonya Sehgal

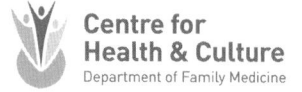
Centre for Health & Culture
Department of Family Medicine

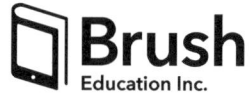
Brush Education Inc.

16 17 18 19 20 5 4 3 2 1

Brush Education Inc.
www.brusheducation.ca
contact@brusheducation.ca

Editorial: Meaghan Craven
Cover and interior design: Carol Dragich, Dragich Design

Printed and manufactured in Canada

Library and Archives Canada Cataloguing in Publication
Waugh, Earle H., 1936–, author
    Cultural competency skills for psychologists, psychotherapists, and counselling professionals : a workbook for caring across cultures / Earle Waugh, Olga Szafran, Jean Triscott, Roger Parent.
Includes bibliographical references.
Issued in print and electronic formats.
ISBN 978-1-55059-652-6 (paperback).—ISBN 978-1-55059-653-3 (pdf).—
ISBN 978-1-55059-654-0 (mobi).—ISBN 978-1-55059-655-7 (epub)

1. Cross-cultural counseling.   2. Minorities—Counseling of.   3. Ethnopsychology.   4. Psychiatry, Transcultural.   I. Szafran, Olga, 1957–, author   II. Triscott, Jean A. C., author   III. Parent, Roger, 1947–, author   IV. Title.

BF636.7.C76W38 2016   158.3089   C2015-905455-9   C2015-905456-7

We acknowledge the support of the Government of Canada.
Nous reconnaissons l'appui du gouvernement du Canada.   Canada

Psychology Team

ROGER GERVAIS has a PhD from the Department of Educational Psychology at the University Alberta. He operates Neurobehavioural Associates.

WES PENNER is a retired counselling psychologist with multiple years counselling and consulting with and for staff and administration in schools, the University of Alberta, and various businesses and institutions across a large part of central and northern Alberta. He asserts that it was his counselling efforts with clients who felt disenfranchised because of religious and cultural differences that refined his ability to empathize with all his clients.

SONYA SEHGAL has an MEd in counselling psychology from the Department of Educational Psychology at the University of Alberta. She is currently a registered provisional psychologist at the Calgary Counselling Centre.

CAROLYN TRISCOTT has an MC from the University of Lethbridge and is a registered psychologist in Alberta.

Contents

Appendices

Preface

Approaches to Culture

Counselling professionals may take many approaches when communicating with clients. The three dominant approaches one sees in the literature are cross-cultural, transcultural, and intercultural. Each of these approaches has a different emphasis on building a bridge with clients.

The theory behind intercultural/multicultural education and training has been under construction since the 1950s and 1960s (Keller, 1989). Many sophisticated models in the literature address cultural issues and are used in the health sciences (Berry, 2011; Denzin & Lincoln, 2005; Geertz, 1973). Critics of the procedures, stances, and social-scientific context of the field have also been many and vigorous (cf. Berube, 2009). Despite the topic's difficulties, this workbook stresses the importance of the multicultural model as an overarching framework and then emphasizes the relational nature of the professional/client encounter through the use of an intercultural approach. The authors of *Cultural Competency Skills for Psychologists, Psychotherapists, and Counselling Professionals* are nevertheless responding to the pressures that exist at the time of this writing to provide practical resources for counselling professionals. We are aware of the objectifying tendency inherent in skill-development processes (Kirmayer, 2012, for example, prefers the transcultural approach), but in our experience, concern with communication in the intercultural context is an acceptable place to begin. Hence, this workbook was written to provide a basic communication model for assisting workers and their managers who confront cultural issues every day in the workplace. In keeping with this basic communication emphasis, we have laboured in both language and concept to make the material accessible. In short, we attempt to provide effective and proven best practices (Bennett, 1998) that will help develop culturally sensitive abilities in counselling professionals today.

REFERENCES

Bennett, M. J. (1998). Intercultural communication: A current perspective. In M. J. Bennett (Ed.), *Basic concepts of intercultural communication: Selected readings* (pp. 1–34).Yarmouth, ME: Intercultural Press.

Berry, J. (2011). Integration and multiculturalism: Ways towards social solidarity. *Papers on Social Representations, 20,* 1–21.

Berube, M. (2009, September 14). What's the matter with cultural studies? *The Chronicle Review.* Retrieved from http://chronicle.com/article/Whats-the-Matter-With/48334

Denzin, N., & Lincoln, Y. S. (Eds.). (2005). *The Sage handbook of qualitative research.* (3rd ed.). Thousand Oaks: Sage Publications.

Geertz, C. (1973). *The interpretation of cultures.* New York: Basic Books.

Keller, D. (1989). *Critical theory, Marxism and modernity.* Cambridge, MA: Polity and John Hopkins University Press.

Kirmayer, L. J. (2012). Rethinking cultural competence. *Transcultural Psychiatry, 49*(2), 149–164. doi:10.1177/1363461512444673

ACKNOWLEDGEMENTS

Two people assisted us with the Muslim section in this workbook: Ms. Lubna Zaeem, BSc (Hons), MEd, who holds a postgraduate certificate in counselling, and Ms. Donna Kampen Entz, BTh, who holds a masters degree in intercultural studies and now works mainly with Southeast Asians in northeast Edmonton.

The authors also wish to acknowledge the ongoing and enthusiastic support they have received from the Department of Family Medicine and its chair, Dr. Lee Green; we especially wish to express appreciation for the work of the staff of the research division in the production of both the manual and this workbook.

This resource also benefits from the excellent work of the many people who contributed to the films that accompany each module. Our thanks go to scriptwriter Mary-Ellen Perley, as well as the Michael Olson and Omar Mouallem filming/directing teams.

Welcome to the Workbook

Purpose

In culturally diverse societies, evidence shows that the beliefs, values, and norms of clients are important factors in the delivery of health care.

Working with people from many cultures is both enriching and challenging. Research in multiple fields has given rise to effective methods and practices for working with people from numerous cultures and for meeting the challenges of cultural diversity. The purpose of this workbook is to make these methods easily accessible and understandable to psychologists.

> In using the term *intercultural*, we emphasize problem solving in bringing people together.

Audience

This workbook is designed specifically for individuals in the counselling professions. Learning tools and high-quality audio-visual resources are used to facilitate the learning process based on real-life situations.

Focus

This workbook approaches culture from the perspective of communication. Rather than trying to describe cultures, the authors focus on understanding the messages and information that are being communicated by clients.

Organization of the Workbook

This workbook offers eight learning modules, two review modules, and one final evaluation. Each of the eight modules contains two parts: a dramatized audio-visual sequence and worksheets. In addition, there are two self-assessments, one at the beginning and another at the end, which allow you to assess your progress.

Outcomes

The skills you acquire through using this workbook will heighten your awareness of cultural issues in health care. You will learn cultural communication and problem-solving skills.

Goal

The goal of this workbook is to help psychologists provide culturally competent care through respectful, effective communication with their clients.

Objectives

This workbook will assist you to:

1. become aware of your own beliefs and attitudes toward clients of different cultural groups;
2. better understand the beliefs and attitudes of your clients;
3. further enhance your skills in intercultural communication and problem solving; and
4. enrich your life-long practice of self-discovery and self-learning in cultural communication.

Modules

In this workbook, we present cultural competency skills in the form of a carefully designed and interrelated sequence of learning modules. Each module presents a real-life scenario that illustrates the challenges you may encounter in the health care setting. The learning tools will assist you to analyze the intercultural situation and find an appropriate solution that is effective and respectful.

Issues

The professionally produced dramatizations in the DVD located at the back of this book illustrate the following range of issues:

- cultural attitudes toward mental health issues (Film: *Depression*),
- cultural issues in obtaining consent (Film: *Informed Consent*),
- cultural issues in compliance (Film: *Machine That Makes Air*),
- language diversity in health care (Film: *Dementia and Language Reversion*),
- modesty codes within cultures (Film: *Modesty Codes and Breast Cancer*),
- post-traumatic stress (Film: *Post-Traumatic Stress*),
- generational views on personal directives (Film: *Living Wills/Personal Directives*),
- challenging cultural norms (Film: *Personal Directive*),
- cultural influence in family decision making (Film: *End-of-Life Issues*),

- traditional roles of family care (Film: *Dementia and Caregiver Stress*), and
- cultural issues in end-of-life care (Film: *No Code*).

> The aim of the dramatizations is to deepen your awareness and insight into the "invisible" language of cultures (beliefs, values, and norms).

Contact Us

If you have any questions, comments, or feedback on the workbook, please contact:

Dr. Earle Waugh, Director
Centre for Health and Culture
Department of Family Medicine
6–10 University Terrace, University of Alberta
Edmonton, Alberta, Canada T6G 2T4
Ph: 780-492-6424, ewaugh@ualberta.ca

Introduction

Diversity: A Reality for All Counselling Professionals

Culture impacts the way in which people perceive the world and how they interact with others. As Canada becomes increasingly multicultural, psychologists working with culturally diverse clients will soon become the norm rather than the exception (Hansen, Pepitone-Arreola-Rockwell, & Greene, 2000). It is therefore necessary to explore the issues that arise when psychologists assist culturally diverse individuals and families. It is important for psychologists and counselling professionals to explore their level of cultural understanding and challenge personal assumptions to demonstrate respect for clients and more fully meet their needs. Blind spots within one's cultural awareness can lead to ineffective treatment and unsuccessful resolution of ethical dilemmas. This manual provides psychologists with practical assessment tools and exercises to help them recognize their level of cultural competence and build upon their skills in an incremental manner. After working through this book, psychologists will be better able to communicate and problem solve with multicultural populations to strengthen the therapeutic working alliance and help their clients overcome barriers.

Psychologists play an important role in addressing cultural complexity. Occupational responsibilities such as counselling, assessment, program development, research, and advocacy are instrumental in shaping the lives of clients and the general population. It can be simple for psychologists to assume that they are culturally sensitive because they strive to be non-judgmental and caring in their approach. However, it is necessary for psychologists to undertake a thorough self-reflective process to determine how their understanding of other cultures impacts the manner in which they interact with others and how others may perceive them based upon their personal characteristics. For example, being a member of the dominant gender or race comes with privileges that are not always immediately visible to those who are part of that dominant group. This manual assists psychologists in asking themselves the questions needed to identify their core beliefs and values within a cultural context.

How should psychologists develop the specific *attitudes*, *knowledge*, and *skills* needed for cultural competence (Collins & Arthur, 2007)? In order for Canadian psychologists to optimize therapeutic outcomes with a wide range of clients from various cultures, culture must be continuously infused into counselling (Collins & Arthur, 2005b). A model that infuses culture into counselling has been developed and is organized according to three core competency domains for the psychologist to learn: (I) cultural awareness of self, (II) cultural awareness of others, and (III) methods of developing a culturally sensitive working alliance (Collins & Arthur, 2007).

Domain I: Cultural awareness of self. Cultural competence is developed when psychologists acknowledge that they are cultural beings with a personal worldview shaped by personal identity, culture, and contextual factors (Arredondo & Glauner, 1992; Sue, 2001). *Personal identity factors* include idiosyncratic experiences, genetic make up, developmental paths, and socialization (Dana, 1998). *Cultural factors* represent the group affiliations held by professionals, including age, gender, ethnicity, physical and mental ability, sexual orientation, religion, language, and social class (Ho, 1995). Lastly, *contextual factors* refer to historical, social, political, environmental, or economic contexts in which professionals live, as these significantly impact personal experiences, worldviews, and values (Arredondo & Glauner, 1992).

Psychologists should undertake self-reflection relative to these factors as each influences how they conceptualize mental health problems and possible solutions, as well as how they choose counselling interventions (Collins & Arthur, 2005b). Moreover, psychologists who remain unaware of their own personal assumptions, values, and biases may create barriers to effective practice with culturally diverse clients (Pedersen, 1995; Ridley, 1995). When working with culturally diverse clients, psychologists can reflect upon their own identity by asking themselves, "What personal, cultural, and contextual factors shape my worldview?" By answering this question honestly, psychologists can bring their authentic selves into the counselling process and remove barriers to effective practice (Collins & Arthur, 2007).

Domain II: Cultural awareness of others. Once you have begun the process of self-reflection on the impact of personal, cultural, and contextual factors on yourself as a person and as a psychologist, you can turn the cultural lens toward the clients you serve. Just as the psychologist's own cultural identity is shaped by historical, social, and cultural experiences and contexts, each client brings with him or her a complex cultural history that affects worldviews, values, assumptions, and beliefs (Arthur & Stewart, 2001; Collins & Arthur, 2005b).

When psychologists become aware of their own cultural assumptions, they require specific (etic) and group-level (emic) knowledge about their clients' cultures. Psychologists can work toward becoming aware of how their own personal identity, cultural, and contextual factors differ from those of their clients. For example, in contrast to having grown up in and perhaps continuing to perpetuate a nuclear family, many clients from different cultures have a collectivist orientation and may reside in intergenerational family structures. Psychologists should also be aware of the relationship of personal culture to health and well-being. This can be done by acknowledging holistic forms of healing and the role of religious and spiritual beliefs in the clients' lives. These beliefs may differ from the Western worldview in the development of psychological problems, expressions of distress, and treatment options (American Psychological Association, 2002).

Although group-level knowledge is important, each culture has significant within-group differences that distinguish individual members of each culture, so psychologists should not assume that all aspects of one culture apply to a particular client until those aspects are directly explored with the individual (Ridley & Kleiner, 2003). When understanding individual differences, psychologists might consider demographic variations in immigration history (reasons for immigration and length of time the family has spent in Canada, for example), as well as social and economic pre- and post-migration experiences (for example, arriving from an urban versus rural background) that shape the lives of clients from different cultures. Psychologists can explore demographics and the cultural identity of their clients by asking, "Who is this client and what aspects of his/her cultural identity are relevant to explore within the counselling context?" (Collins & Arthur, 2007; Ho, 1995).

Psychologists should also aim to find a balance between never applying cultural knowledge and assuming that all psychological problems are influenced by cultural factors (Collins & Arthur, 2005b; Pedersen, 1995). Furthermore, psychologists can learn how to recognize which aspects of cultural identity are relevant to explore by opening their eyes to *cultural blindness*: the belief that no difference exists between people (Cross, Bazron, Dennis & Isaacs, 1989). Psychologists can move away from this position by becoming aware of differences and fostering acceptance and respect for them (Cross et al., 1989).

Domain III: Culturally sensitive working alliance. The working alliance between the psychologist and the client is a key factor to therapeutic success (Shapiro, 1995) and is composed of three core components: (a) trust and respect, (b) agreement on goals, and (c) agreement on tasks (Collins & Arthur, 2005a). The point of connection between the psychologist's awareness of self (Domain I) and awareness of the cultural identity of the client (Domain II) leads to what is known as a culturally sensitive working alliance. Establishing a working alliance across cultures requires reconciliation between the Western worldview and differing beliefs and can be a challenging process.

To build trust and respect, psychologists are encouraged to engage in cultural exploration with their clients regarding attitudes toward counselling. Any cultural mistrust and value disconnects between psychologists and clients can also be explored, as differences between Western and other worldviews can affect beliefs about seeing a psychologist and follow-through with interventions. Psychologists may also need to be flexible in the way they communicate (Sue & Sue, 1999), office setting, times for counselling appointments, and expectations implicit for the roles of psychologist and client (Amundson, 1998).

A culturally sensitive working alliance also includes psychologist–client collaboration in establishing goals that are responsive to salient dimensions of the client's cultural identity. Since cultural identity impacts how both the psychologist and the client understand appropriate targets for change (APA, 2002), failure to understand cultural dynamics may result in a mismatch between psychologist and client in counselling goals and premature termination of counselling (Collins & Arthur, 2005a). When working toward building a culturally sensitive working alliance, psychologists can ask themselves, "Whose agenda is driving the counselling process and how might I ensure that the goals we have established are not biased by my own beliefs or values about success in counselling?" (Collins & Arthur, 2007).

Once psychologists and clients have agreed on goals, the last step is to collaborate on developing counselling interventions that are culturally sensitive (Collins & Arthur, 2005a). Depending on the nature of the mental health concern(s) and the salience of cultural factors to the goals of counselling, psychologists may need to draw on a wide range of interventions, including professional consultation, training, and planning strategies that are culturally competent (Collins & Arthur, 2005a).

We employ practical examples in this manual to illustrate several clinical situations that may test a psychologist's level of cultural competency. Psychologists are given the opportunity to work through these clinical situations step-by-step and thoroughly explore the cultural dilemmas depicted. The more experience psychologists gain visualizing the clinical scenario, the more likely they will be able to address it with confidence. Psychologists must practice skills related to these scenarios in order to successfully integrate them into their repertoire. This applied method of learning allows psychologists to work at their own pace and ask questions that influence further development.

It is important to note that increasing the level of cultural competency is a reflexive practice. It is essential to recognize how clients impact psychologists and how psychologists impact their clients, in turn. Each individual brings a rich history of tradition, rituals, and ways of being into the therapeutic setting. If psychologists can learn how to address similarities and differences in an open manner, they allow for a greater level of trust and empathy in their dealings with clients. The invisible elephant in the room must be addressed in order for psychologists to successfully establish working relationships and promote a greater level of hope and well-being. Thus, this manual provides psychologists with a vehicle and starting point to explore the process of cultural competence.

Understanding Culture

Definitions of Culture

No single definition of culture has been accepted by all health care professionals. The learning activities and resources in this workbook are based on the view that culture consists of "our routine actions, our interpretations of meanings in those actions, and in the beliefs that underlie our interpretations" (Banks & Banks, 2010, p. 35). The interpretations of meanings are further examined in light of individual beliefs, values, and norms. Elements of culture include language, religion, customs, and traditions, family roles and relationships, food, clothing, and arts and literature, among others.

The Cultural Backbone: Beliefs, Values, and Norms

A culture, as well as its individual members, may communicate in a specific and invisible way and with a particular cultural viewpoint. Viewpoints encompass the beliefs, values, and norms of a particular culture.

Belief: A point of view that the individual deems to be true or false.

Value: An individual's sense of right and wrong concerning an appropriate course of action or outcome.

Norm: An individual's pattern of behaviours in an everyday context. *Social norms* are how a group expects an individual to behave in a given context.

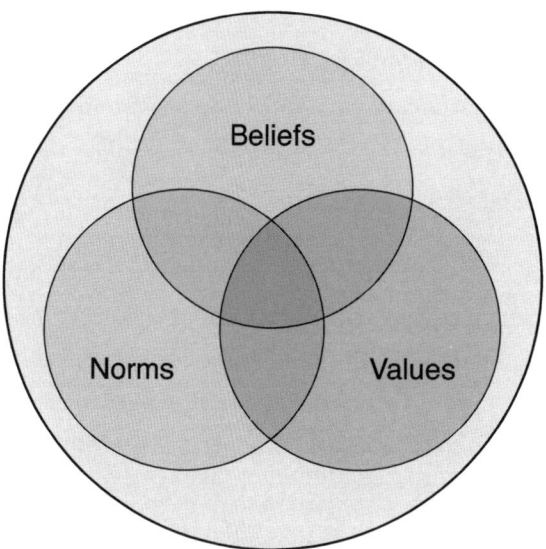

Figure 1: Culture is a combination of beliefs, values, and norms.

....

The Importance of Cultural Competency Training

Counselling professionals are faced with the challenge of caring for clients from many cultures, with different languages, varying socio-economic status, and different understandings of illness and health, all of which can affect the amount and kind of care clients receive. Culture is a predominant force in shaping behaviour, values, and institutions. Cultural differences between clients and counselling professionals may affect health care delivery and the counselling relationship.

Research has shown that ethno-cultural health and disease belief systems affect client–provider interactions (Harwood, 1981; Hill, 1976; Kleinman, Eisenberg, and Good, 1978; Martinez, 1978; Mason, 1980; Muecke, 1983; Snow, 1974). With immigrant populations and diversity becoming ever more a reality the world over, it is evident that the cultural landscape will continue to be a factor in the provision of health care.

Cultural Competency Skills for Psychologists, Psychotherapists, and Counselling Professionals

The development of cultural competency skills has become a necessity for psychologists. Lack of cultural knowledge on the part of psychologists has been associated with improper diagnoses (Faison & Mintzer, 2005), lack of active compliance (Sattar, et al., 2004), social resistance (Opolka, Rascati, Brown and Gibson, 2004), and legal challenges (Beauchamp, 2007a, 2007b; Guichon, 2007).

The cultural orientation of counselling professionals can influence access and use of health services by various cultural groups. Ethno-cultural factors affect the amount and type of care individuals belonging to various cultural groups receive (Daker-White, Beattie, Gilliard, and Means, 2002); therefore, cultural competency has the potential to reduce inequities.

Both quality of care and the detection of culturally specific diseases have been shown to increase with the provision of culturally sensitive health care. Cultural competency improves both the client–provider relationship and health professional communication with clients (Betancourt, Green, Carrillo, and Park, 2005).

Counselling professionals can develop the ability to interact and intervene among diverse ethno-cultural groups with sensitivity, knowledge, and skill (Lum, 1992)—in other words, with cultural competence. Cultural competence enables health care providers to assist clients from various ethno-cultural groups in useful and acceptable ways that are consistent with clients' values, beliefs, and expectations (Gallagher-Thompson, Talamantes, Ramirez, and Valverde, 1996).

Cultural competency has been defined as "a set of congruent behaviors, attitudes, and policies that come together in a system, agency, or amongst professionals and enables that system, agency, or those professionals to work effectively in cross-cultural situations" (Cross, Bazron, Dennis, and Isaacs, 1989).

Cultural competency is the:

> acceptance and respect for difference, continuing self-assessment regarding culture, careful attention to the dynamics of difference, continuous expansion of cultural knowledge and resources, and a variety of adaptations to service models in order to better meet the needs of minority populations. (Cross et al., 1989)

It is also the "ability to think, feel and act in ways that acknowledge, respect, and build upon ethnic, (socio) cultural, and linguistic diversity" (Lynch & Hanson, 1998).

The goals of culturally competent care are to "create a health care system and workforce that are capable of delivering the highest-quality care to every client regardless of race, ethnicity, culture, or language proficiency" (Betancourt et al., 2005).

Culturally competent counselling professionals have the ability to understand, communicate with, and effectively interact with people of different cultures. They are not threatened by another culture's perspective but rather welcome collaboration and co-operation.

> The development of cultural competence requires training and education, and it takes time. It is a dynamic and continuous process of life-long learning.

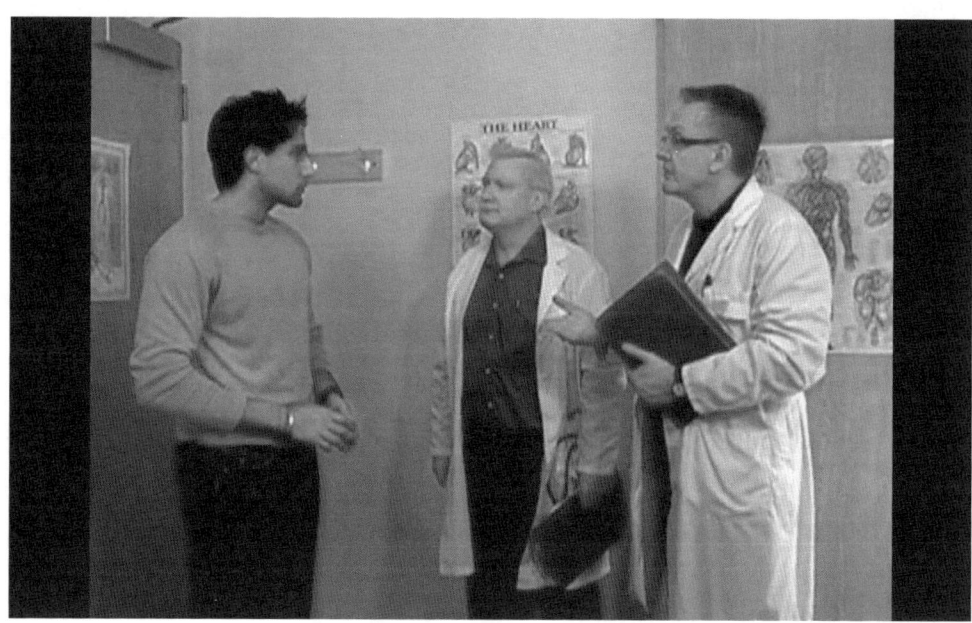

Communicating Across Cultures

In the client-counsellor encounter, the client has a cultural perspective; at the same time, the counselling professional has a personal cultural stance, as well as a professional cultural perspective. Intercultural communication occurs when common ground is reached between the health professional and client (see Figure 2). Common ground is something people agree on even if they disagree about other things. Reaching common ground lays the foundation for mutual understanding and enables the client and health care team to move forward in providing care that is in the best interest of the client.

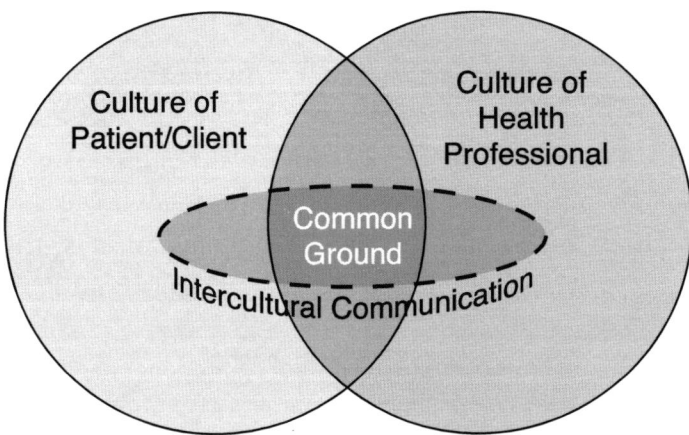

Figure 2: Model of Intercultural Communication

Beliefs and attitudes about health services vary greatly among different cultures. Therefore, it is essential to build trust and respect with each client and the client's community. Culturally competent care respects beliefs, values, behaviours, daily practices, language, communication styles, attire, food, reaction to pain, and cultural decision-making styles. Trust and respect are gained through communication. When psychologists and counselling professionals communicate across cultures, they are building a bridge with the client.

The Metaphor of the Bridge to Help with Communication

To help you understand cultural relationships, we use the metaphor of building a bridge. This bridge is communication. Communicating effectively with a person from a different culture means being able to understand the culture's norms, values, and beliefs.

These norms, values, and beliefs, are shared by specific groups, and they can differ from your own. Recognizing another culture's norms, values, and beliefs allows you to understand how different groups have distinct ways of understanding everyday life. These different ways of understanding impact families, institutions, organizations, and systems. This workbook will help you build a bridge of cultural communication by learning to recognize cultural norms, values, and beliefs.

Building a Cultural Competency Bridge

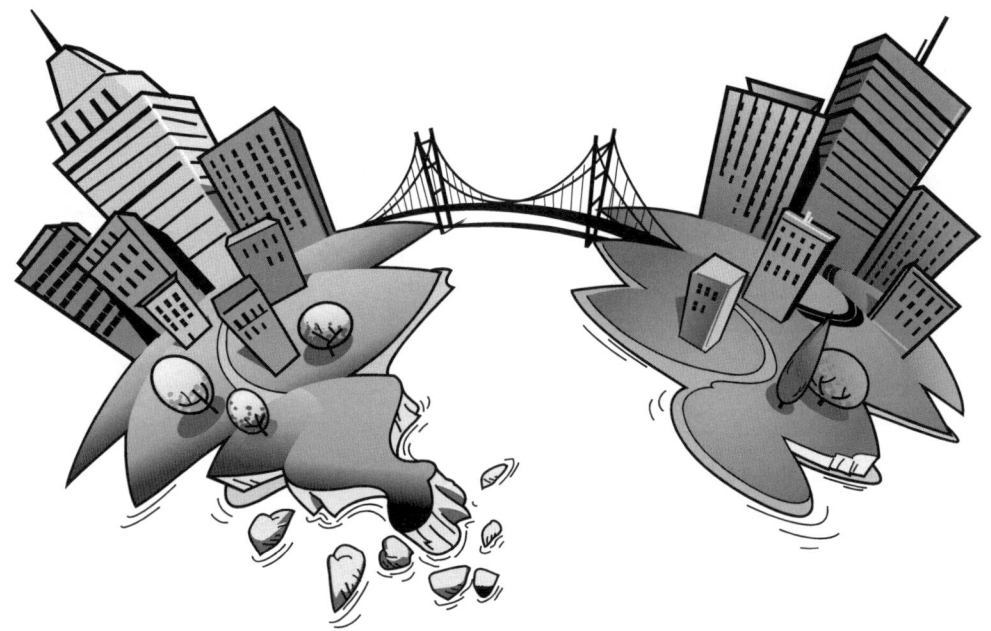

© iStock.com/soberve

Different cultural communities can be thought of as islands in the sea. Psychologists and counselling professionals, of course, belong to their own cultural communities, which may be different from those of their clients. In order for both of these cultural and professional communities to communicate, they need to find a common understanding; they need to build a bridge. Building a cultural competency bridge is a way to reach common ground (Figure 3).

The better the bridge, the better the communication. Communication on the bridge goes both ways. For the health professional, building a competency bridge is necessary to provide respectful client care.

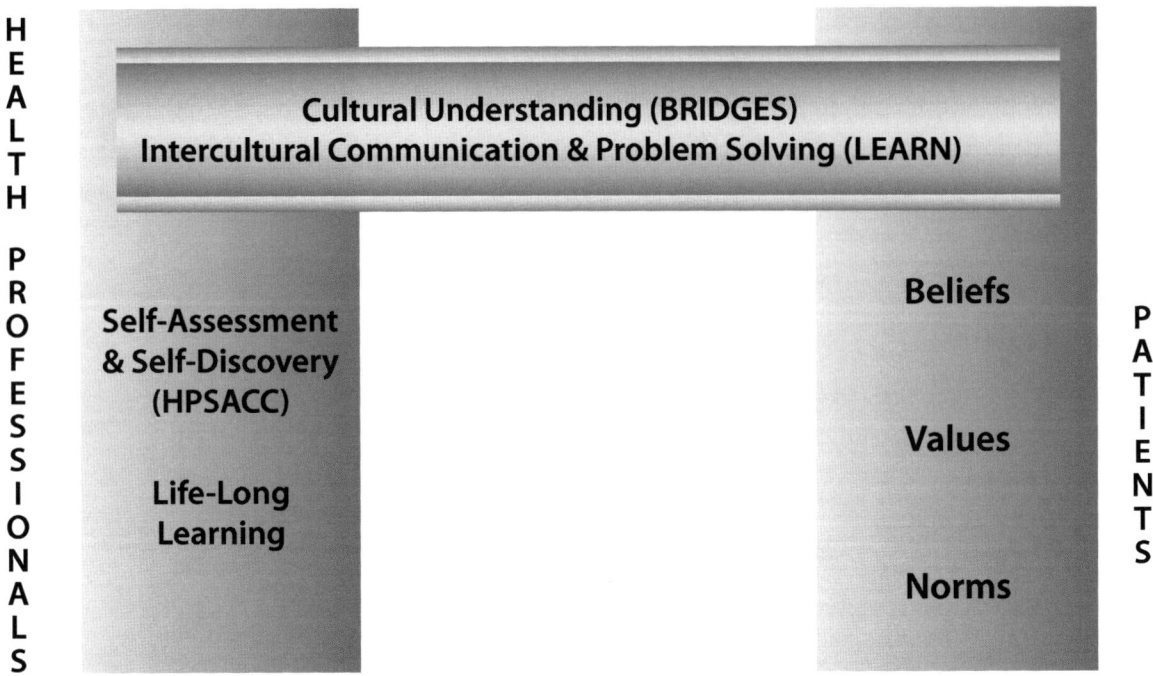

Figure 3: Tools for Building a Cultural Competency Bridge

How to Build Bridges with Clients

Psychologists and counselling professionals communicate with clients every day, but communication is not just speaking a common language. Communication takes on many other forms. When counselling professionals become aware of client beliefs, values, and norms, they find that they can communicate more effectively with clients about health issues. Counselling professionals use a variety of communication techniques that are not language specific, including:

1. *Non-verbal Language* Facial expressions and body gestures can say more than words and often be more informative than spoken words.

2. *Communication Customs* Effective use of customs can ease rapport, such as shaking hands at introduction, keeping an acceptable space between each other, and maintaining culturally appropriate eye contact during conversation.

3. *Verbal Language* Spoken words can contain hidden messages, and often the real meaning behind spoken words are never said.

4. *Attitudes* Attitudes can reflect certain cultural perspectives; learning cultural attitudes will provide a foundation for communication.

5. *Use of Idioms* All cultures have idioms that refer to common experiences and are a kind of short-hand way of speaking about an issue. Learning some of these can be a helpful way to communicate.

6. *Use of Humour* Humour can "break the ice" quicker than serious talk; a culturally appropriate joke can unite teller and listener in personal ways so that more serious issues are easier to discuss.

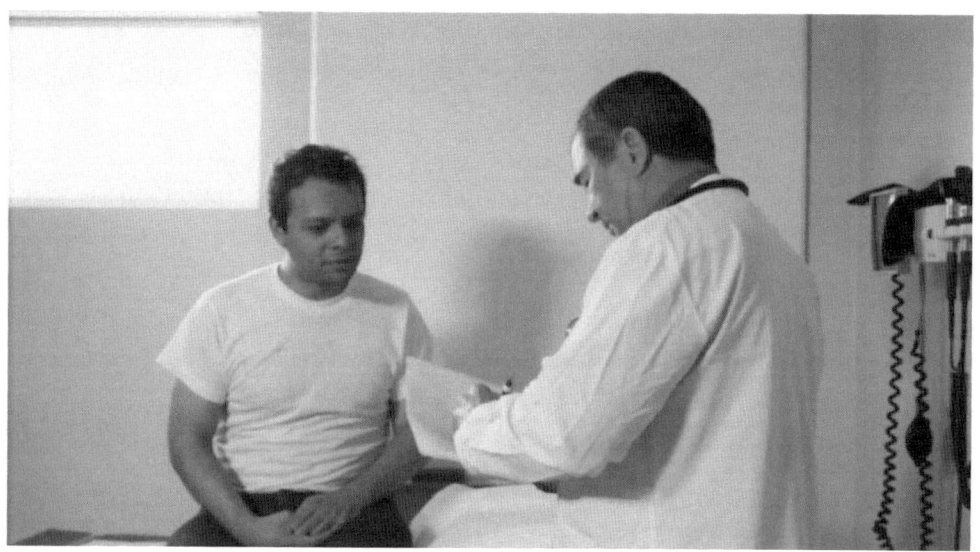

. . . .

Tools to Building a Cultural Competency Bridge

Four elements to developing cultural competency skills include:

1. the process of self-assessment and self-discovery;

2. developing a cultural understanding of the client's perspective;

3. developing skills in intercultural communication; and

4. self-directed, life-long learning.

Tools are available to assist you in developing skills in each of these elements. A discussion of these tools follows.

The Health Professional's Self-Assessment of Cultural Competency (HPSACC) Questionnaire (Psychology Version)

Self-assessment and self-discovery is a process of gaining insight into your own beliefs, values, and attitudes (Mason, 1996). Becoming aware of how these influence your personal and professional relationships will provide the foundations for working in a positive, intercultural manner.

The Health Professional's Self-Assessment of Cultural Competency (HPSACC) Questionnaire (Psychology Version) (Waugh, Szafran, and Hanafi, 2011) was developed by our team to help health care professionals evaluate their own cultural knowledge, awareness, sensitivity, behaviours, and cultural confidence. We revised our original HPSACC Questionnaire to develop a psychology version. The HPSACC (Psychology Version) is designed to assess the components necessary in a professional to produce culturally competent care. Culturally competent care is that in which the efficacy of the interaction between the client and the professional is not hindered by cultural elements, such that health outcomes are improved, costs are lowered, and client compliance is increased. Competency is personal ability that allows a person to function effectively. The purpose of this self-assessment is to encourage counselling professionals to reflect on their ability to deliver culturally competent care and recognize areas for growth and improvement. The goal is to sensitize psychologists and counsellors to the need for culturally competent care and induce a desire to develop the ability to deliver such care.

Work through the following questions, taking time to reflect on your personal and professional cultural perspectives. There are six sections, each one dealing with a distinctive aspect of cultural competency. Using the rating scale located on the right, indicate the number that adequately describes your awareness of each item. After you have completed the questionnaire, reflect on your strengths and the areas in which you would like to improve. After you have completed the workbook, please redo the HPSACC Question-naire and observe any changes that have occurred.

The Health Professional's Self-Assessment of Cultural Competency (HPSACC) Questionnaire (Psychology Version)

For each of the following questions, circle the number under "Rating" that most accurately describes you.

1. To what extent do you **AGREE** with each of the following statements?

1 = strongly disagree, 2 = moderately disagree, 3 = slightly disagree 4 = slightly agree, 5 = moderately agree, 6 = strongly agree	Rating (circle one)					
a) I have had many *cross-cultural encounters in my life.*	1	2	3	4	5	6
b) I frequently *take part in cross-cultural interactions.*	1	2	3	4	5	6
c) I encounter people from a wide *variety of cultural groups.*	1	2	3	4	5	6
d) I partake in comprehensive *and in-depth cross-cultural interactions.*	1	2	3	4	5	6
e) In general, my cross-cultural encounters have been positive *experiences.*	1	2	3	4	5	6

2. How **INFORMED** are you about each of the following areas for the community that you serve?

1 = highly uninformed, 2 = moderately uninformed, 3 = slightly uninformed, 4 = slightly informed, 5 = moderately informed, 6 = highly informed, NA = does not apply	Rating (circle one)					
a) demographic data describing the cultural groups you serve (age, income, education, etc.)	1	2	3	4	5	6
b) social and cultural characteristics of the cultural groups you serve	1	2	3	4	5	6
c) different food choices/habits of the cultural groups you serve	1	2	3	4	5	6
d) different physical activity practices of the cultural groups you serve	1	2	3	4	5	6
e) different spiritual/faith practices of the cultural groups you serve	1	2	3	4	5	6
f) different ideas of family roles in the cultural groups you serve	1	2	3	4	5	6
g) different attitudes about the Western model of illness within the cultural groups you serve	1	2	3	4	5	6
h) different healing traditions/methods (Ayurvedic medicine, traditional Chinese medicine, etc.) of the cultural groups you serve	1	2	3	4	5	6
i) different methods and behaviours of seeking help for health issues in the cultural groups you serve	1	2	3	4	5	6
j) different factors that increase or reduce risk to illness (smoking, availability of social support, etc.) that are predominant in the cultural groups you serve	1	2	3	4	5	6
k) differences in health status (life expectancy, mortality rates, etc.) that are predominant in the cultural groups you serve	1	2	3	4	5	6
l) health disparities (access to health care, health outcomes, etc.) that are predominant in the cultural groups you serve	1	2	3	4	5	6

1 = highly uninformed, 2 = moderately uninformed, 3 = slightly uninformed, 4 = slightly informed, 5 = moderately informed, 6 = highly informed, NA = does not apply	Rating (circle one)					
m) how different cultural groups vary in their responses to medications(ethnopharmacology)	1	2	3	4	5	6
n) government (local, regional, national) policies dealing with multiculturalism	1	2	3	4	5	6
o) your organization's policy on the subject of multiculturalism NA	1	2	3	4	5	6

3. How **AWARE** are you of each of the following areas of transcultural interaction?

1 = highly unaware, 2 = moderately unaware, 3 = slightly unaware 4 = slightly aware, 5 = moderately aware, 6 = highly aware	Rating (circle one)					
a) your own cultural identity (including professional culture) and how this affects your interactions with clients	1	2	3	4	5	6
b) differences in views and attitudes within your own cultural group	1	2	3	4	5	6
c) your own cultural stereotypes and how these affect your interactions with clients	1	2	3	4	5	6
d) your own biases/prejudices and how these affect your interactions with clients	1	2	3	4	5	6
e) beliefs and values of the organization you work for and how these affect clients	1	2	3	4	5	6
f) significant similarities and differences between the cultural groups in the community that you serve	1	2	3	4	5	6
g) variation among people belonging to one cultural group	1	2	3	4	5	6
h) the possibility that a person may identify with more than one cultural group	1	2	3	4	5	6
i) the influence of many cultural aspects on health and health care	1	2	3	4	5	6

4. To what extent do you **AGREE** with each of the following statements?

1 = strongly disagree, 2 = moderately disagree, 3 = slightly disagree 4 = slightly agree, 5 = moderately agree, 6 = strongly agree	Rating (circle one)					
a) I feel that cultural beliefs and differences should be respected and accepted.	1	2	3	4	5	6
b) I think all clients should be treated with respect, no matter their culture.	1	2	3	4	5	6
c) I believe that psychologists and counsellors should be caring and considerate of clients and their needs.	1	2	3	4	5	6
d) I feel that psychologists and counsellors should approach clients with humility.	1	2	3	4	5	6
e) I regard trust as an important part of a psychologist's/counsellor's relationship with the client.	1	2	3	4	5	6
f) I believe that knowledge of cultural groups helps guide a psychologist's/ counsellor's work with clients.	1	2	3	4	5	6
g) I think that no matter how much knowledge a professional believes s/he has about a client's culture, s/he must still assess the client's personal preference for offered services.	1	2	3	4	5	6
h) I believe it is important for professionals to learn about cultural competency.	1	2	3	4	5	6

5. How **SKILLED** do you feel in each of the following areas of transcultural interaction?

1 = highly unskilled, 2 = moderately unskilled, 3 = slightly unskilled
4 = slightly skilled, 5 = moderately skilled, 6 = highly skilled
NA = does not apply

If the behaviour applies to your profession, indicate how **FREQUENTLY** you demonstrate each behaviour when the opportunity presents itself.

1 = never (less than 10% of the time)	*2 = almost never (11–25% of the time)*	*3 = sometimes (26–50% of the time)*
4 = often (51–75% of the time)	*5 = almost always (76–90% of the time)*	*6 = always (more than 90% of the time)*

	SKILL	FREQUENCY
a) using a variety of resources to help you learn more about people from different cultures	1 2 3 4 5 6 NA	1 2 3 4 5 6
b) documenting cultural factors and cultural issues that arise when you interact with clients	1 2 3 4 5 6 NA	1 2 3 4 5 6
c) documenting adjustments to care that you make for clients' cultural needs	1 2 3 4 5 6 NA	1 2 3 4 5 6
d) greeting clients in a culturally appropriate way	1 2 3 4 5 6 NA	1 2 3 4 5 6
e) apologizing for cross-cultural misunderstandings or errors	1 2 3 4 5 6 NA	1 2 3 4 5 6
f) asking clients for cultural feedback about the care you have provided	1 2 3 4 5 6 NA	1 2 3 4 5 6
g) asking clients about their general beliefs about health	1 2 3 4 5 6 NA	1 2 3 4 5 6
h) asking clients about their views of the specific health issue at hand (its cause, name, treatment, course, probable outcome, chances of recovery, etc.)	1 2 3 4 5 6 NA	1 2 3 4 5 6
i) identifying clients' expectations for care	1 2 3 4 5 6 NA	1 2 3 4 5 6
j) addressing clients' use of folk remedies and/or alternative healing methods (Ayurvedic medicine, traditional Chinese medicine, etc.)	1 2 3 4 5 6 NA	1 2 3 4 5 6
k) addressing clients' use of folk healers and/or alternative health practitioners (shaman, medicine man, acupuncturist, etc.)	1 2 3 4 5 6 NA	1 2 3 4 5 6
l) assessing clients' ability to understand health-related information (health literacy)	1 2 3 4 5 6 NA	1 2 3 4 5 6
m) learning and using keywords to communicate with specific cultural groups in the community that you serve	1 2 3 4 5 6 NA	1 2 3 4 5 6
n) using a professional interpreter to facilitate effective communication when necessary	1 2 3 4 5 6 NA	1 2 3 4 5 6

1 = never (less than 10% of the time)	2 = almost never (11–25% of the time)	3 = sometimes (26–50% of the time)
4 = often (51–75% of the time)	5 = almost always (76–90% of the time)	6 = always (more than 90% of the time)

	SKILL	FREQUENCY
o) modifying client health-education materials and/ or techniques to meet the cultural needs of your clients	1 2 3 4 5 6 NA	1 2 3 4 5 6
p) explaining procedures, results, and options to clients at an appropriate level for their understanding	1 2 3 4 5 6 NA	1 2 3 4 5 6
q) performing culturally sensitive tests	1 2 3 4 5 6 NA	1 2 3 4 5 6
r) negotiating treatment plans and/or referrals according to the cultural needs of clients	1 2 3 4 5 6 NA	1 2 3 4 5 6
s) dealing with clients who do not follow the recommended course of treatment (adherence/ compliance problems)	1 2 3 4 5 6 NA	1 2 3 4 5 6
t) providing culturally appropriate end-of-life counselling	1 2 3 4 5 6 NA	1 2 3 4 5 6
u) dealing with cross-cultural conflict in interactions with clients	1 2 3 4 5 6 NA	1 2 3 4 5 6

6. To what extent do you **AGREE** with each of the following statements?

1 = strongly disagree, 2 = moderately disagree, 3 = slightly disagree 4 = slightly agree, 5 = moderately agree, 6 = strongly agree	Rating (circle one)					
a) I am comfortable interacting with clients of a different culture.	1	2	3	4	5	6
b) I am confident in my knowledge of areas of cross-cultural interaction.	1	2	3	4	5	6
c) I am self-assured in my awareness of areas of cross-cultural interaction.	1	2	3	4	5	6
d) I am certain that I am sensitive to issues of cross-cultural interaction.	1	2	3	4	5	6
e) I am confident in my ability to use culturally competent behaviours in interactions with clients.	1	2	3	4	5	6
f) I am satisfied with the culturally competent care I provide to clients.	1	2	3	4	5	6

7. How much training in cultural diversity or cultural competency do you **DESIRE** to receive? (*circle one*)

1 = none	2 = a little	3 = some	4 = quite a bit	5 = a lot

Thank you for your time and effort completing the questionnaire.

Developing Cultural Understanding (BRIDGES Tool)

Culture comprises many different elements. To develop cultural understanding, we need to be aware of each of these elements. Cultural understanding is being aware that there are differences in people's worldviews. Gaining an understanding of clients' cultural perspectives is important to reach common ground. To assist you in developing cultural understanding, we suggest using BRIDGES in a deeper way—as an acronym or a tool to help you recall the elements of culture. Remembering it will assist you when eliciting important information about your clients' cultural perspectives. We provide some suggested questions below to assist you.

Beliefs, values, norms

What do you believe the origin of this health issue to be?
What cultural aspect do you value the most in your current situation?
What would normally be done in this situation in your culture?

Roles and relationships with family/relatives

What is your family situation?
What role do you play in your family or community?
What roles do each of your family members have in regard to your illness?

Identify language, literacy, communication

What language do you feel most comfortable speaking?
What is your highest level of education?

Decision-making methods/practices

How are decisions normally made in your family?
Who is involved in family decision making?

Group, community, organizations

What cultural group do you normally associate with?
What faith group do you belong to or identify with?

Extraordinary issues in health (end-of-life, childbirth, etc.)

Are there certain cultural practices associated with your health issue (at end-of-life, or in a crisis) in your community?

Share understanding of cultures, reach common ground, and compromise

How do you think we differ on this health issue? How are we similar? What do you think we have in common?

Intercultural Communication (LEARN Model)

Intercultural communication is the key to developing shared understandings and mutually agreed-upon solutions. Developed by Berlin and Fowkes (1983), the LEARN Model is a set of guidelines that improve communication between counselling professionals and clients during intercultural encounters. The LEARN Model is a tool that will facilitate the provision of culturally sensitive care that is client-centred, avoids stereotyping, and leads to an adoption of mutually acceptable care and/or treatment decisions. The LEARN Model helps develop communication and problem-solving skills to reach common ground.

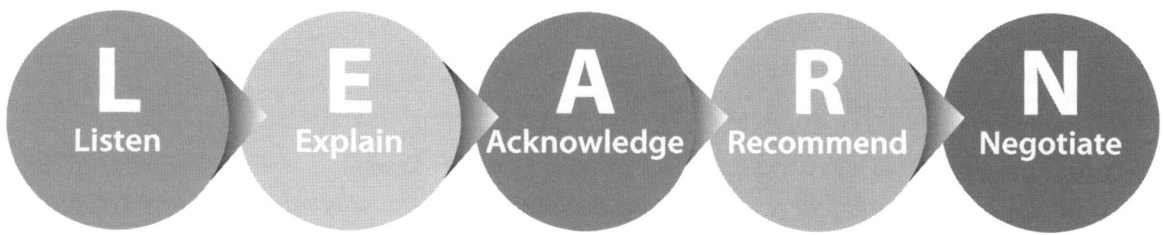

L*isten with cultural sensitivity, aware of your client/clients' cultural perspective.*

E*xplain your perspective of the health issue.*

A*cknowledge differences/similarities with your clients.*

R*ecommend treatment respectfully and sensitively.*

N*egotiate an agreement with your client and his or her family or caregiver.*

Listen *to the client's perception of the cause, process, duration, and outcome of an illness, as well as healing strategies and resources that the client considers to be appropriate.*

Helpful questions: What do you feel may be causing your problem? How do you feel the illness is affecting you? What do you feel might be of benefit?

Explain *your perception of the problem to the client. Most often, this is a biomedical explanation of your (the provider's) best-educated analysis.*

Helpful tips: Use simple language. Avoid medical jargon. Confirm that the client understands the problem as explained.

Acknowledge *the client's explanation and understanding of the illness. Acknowledgement of both the client's and provider's explanatory models of illness will identify areas of agreement and lead to resolution of potential conceptual conflicts between different belief systems.*

Helpful questions: What do you call your problem? When did it start? What do you think caused the problem? Have you taken any medicines or herbs? What results have you had? Do you believe the illness is serious? How can I help you? (Kleinman, 1981)

Recommend *a treatment plan that involves the client in the planning. When appropriate, include culturally relevant approaches to increase the client's acceptance of the treatment plan.*

Key point: Be sensitive to the cultural implications of the treatment plan. It is important to use culturally appropriate wording when explaining the plan to the client.

Negotiate *the client's agreement to the treatment plan by incorporating the client's cultural framework of health and healing with the provider's medical recommendations. Both the client and provider are part of this decision-making process.*

Helpful questions: Is there a culturally appropriate way we can make the treatment plan work for you? Who do you want to be included in your care and medical decisions?

In the next chapter, you will use the LEARN Model and BRIDGES Tool to work through Modules 1 through 8.

Tips for Cultural Communication

Below are several tips that will help you communicate with clients in a respectful, effective manner concerning culturally sensitive health issues. Counselling professionals can use these every day to reach common ground with clients.

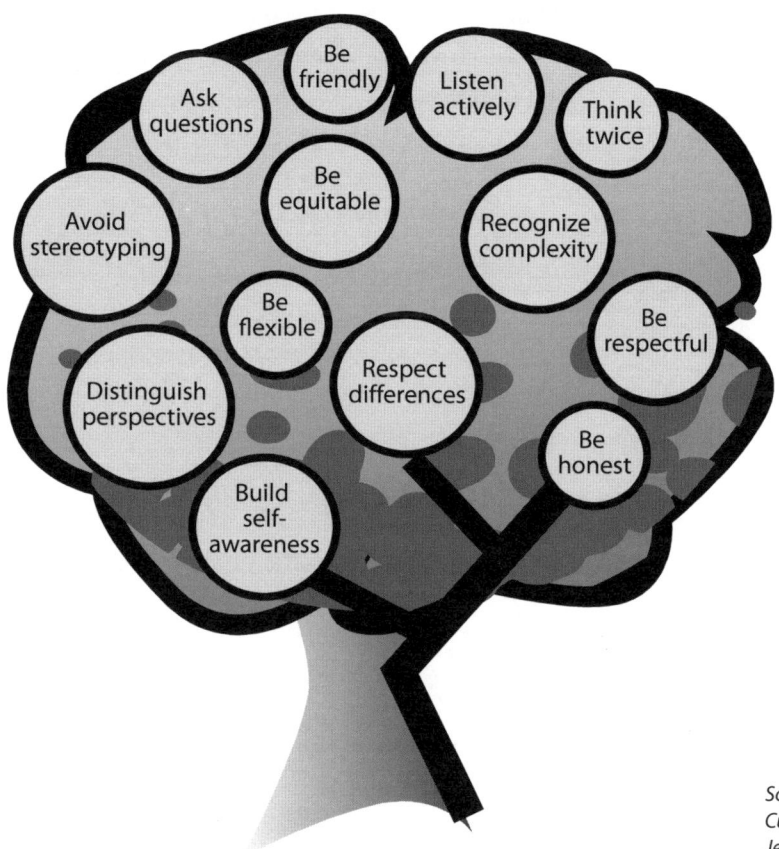

Source: Adapted from "Ten Strategies for Cross-Cultural Communication" by the New York New Jersey Public Health Training Center (2004).

Listen Actively	Be aware of the concerns behind the responses.
Respect Differences	Appreciation of various life-paths reaps big rewards.
Avoid Stereotyping	Despite their group identity, individuals see things differently.
Recognize Complexity	Families and relationships are never simple.
Build Self-Awareness	Use your experience in health care to build your own awareness skills.
Distinguish Perspectives	Everyone tries to protect their own view of things.
Ask Questions	Better to ask than to decide based on too little information.
Think Twice	Stand in the client's shoes and resist quick decisions.
Be Flexible	Admit that boundaries of protocol can limit health care solutions.
Be Honest	Clients need to know that solutions are not easy.

Life-Long Learning

Life-long learning is defined as "all learning activity undertaken throughout life, with the aim of improving knowledge, skills and competences within a personal, civic, social and/or employment-related perspective" (Commission of European Communities, 2001).

Learning can be seen as something that takes place on an ongoing basis as a result of our daily interactions with others and with the world around us. No one becomes an expert instantly. Life-long learning is ongoing and voluntary. The development of cultural competency skills is a dynamic and continuous process that occurs throughout one's professional and personal life.

Organizations and individuals must be able to adjust and enhance their knowledge and skills to meet evolving health needs. Health professions, in particular, are developing practitioners to be life-long learners.

Life-long learning will assist you in developing skills in self-reflection and critical thinking. It can take the form of formal, informal, or self-directed learning.

Strategies for life-long learning may include the following items.

1. Cultural Case Studies

Cultural case studies are examples of interactions from your own experience that directly express the role of culture. Such a case study may have an ethnic, religious, or distinctive cultural foundation. Try to analyze such experiences by applying the LEARN and BRIDGES tools and share them with your colleagues. A portfolio of these case studies is helpful for discussions related to cultural competence. Take care that the people in the examples remain anonymous, and respect confidentiality issues.

2. Small-Group, Problem-Based Learning (SGPBL)

Small-group, problem-based learning (SGPBL) is learner centred and conducted in small groups of six to ten people. The cultural problem forms the basis of the learning and is a vehicle for the development of problem-solving skills. The process is guided by a group facilitator. In the workplace, SGPBL can be part of continuing professional development.

3. Participate in Professional Development on Cultural Competency

All psychologists and counselling professionals are required to keep up-to-date on and participate in professional development. Professional development may include:
(a) attending lectures, conferences, and/or workshops on cultural issues in health;
(b) consulting experts on a cultural issue or a particular case; and/or (c) pursuing higher-level education.

4. Expanding Personal Cultural Experiences

Each person lives in a particular cultural environment, and insights gained from personal experiences influence professional perspectives. In a multicultural work environment, it is necessary to expand one's cultural perspectives. This can be achieved by associating with people from other cultural backgrounds, attending cultural events, travelling, and learning another language.

5. Learning Resources

Many cultural learning resources are available in print and on the Internet. Some are listed in this workbook.

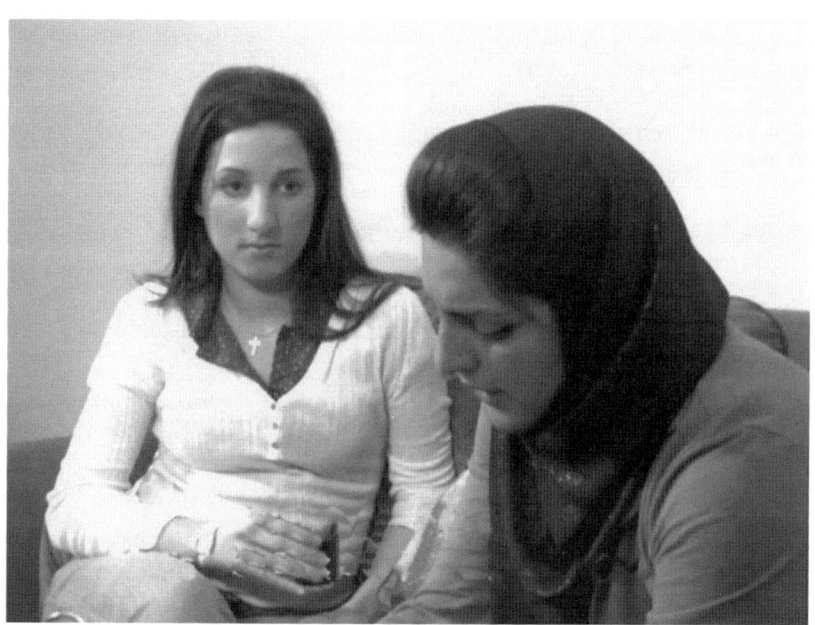

REFERENCES

Amundson, N. E. (1998). *Active engagement: Enhancing the career counselling process*. Richmond, BC: Ergon Communications.

Arredondo, P., & Glauner, T. (1992). *Personal dimensions of identity model*. Boston, MA: Empowerment Workshops.

Arthur, N., & Stewart, J. (2001). Multicultural counselling in the new millennium: Introduction to the special theme issue. *Canadian Journal of Counselling, 35*(1), 3–14.

Banks, J. A., & Banks, M. C. A. (2010). *Multicultural education: Issues and perspectives* (7th ed.). Needham Heights, MA: Allyn & Bacon.

Beauchamp, P. (2007a, November 24). Court fight saved man's life, family says. Do-not-resuscitate order fought. *Calgary Herald*, A1.

Beauchamp, P. (2007b, December 30). No regrets over court fight for fall victim's family. Calgary senior on road to recovery after coma. *Calgary Herald*, B3.

Berlin, E. A., & Fowkes, W. (1983). A teaching framework for cross-cultural health care: Application in family practice. *Western Journal of Medicine, 139*(6), 934–938.

Betancourt, J. R., Green, A. R., Carrillo, J. E., & Park, E. R. (2005). Cultural competence and health care disparities: Key perspectives and trends. *Health Affairs, 24*(2), 499–505. http://dx.doi.org/10.1377/hlthaff.24.2.499

Collins, S., & Arthur, N. (2005a). Enhancing the therapeutic alliance in culture-infused counselling. In N. Arthur & S. Collins (Eds.), *Culture-infused counselling: Celebrating the Canadian mosaic* (pp. 103–149). Calgary, AB: Counselling Concepts.

Collins, S., & Arthur, N. (2005b). Multicultural counselling competencies: A framework for professional development. In N. Arthur & S. Collins (Eds.), *Culture-infused counselling: Celebrating the Canadian mosaic* (pp. 41–102). Calgary, AB: Counselling Concepts.

Collins, S., & Arthur, N. (2007). A framework for enhancing multicultural counselling competence. *Canadian Journal of Counselling, 41*(1), 31–49.

Commission of European Communities (2001, November 21). *Making a European area of lifelong learning a reality* (Communication from the Commission, COM[2001] 678 final). Retrieved October 22, 2014, from http://eur-lex .europa.eu/LexUriServ/LexUriServ.do?uri=COM:2001:0678:FIN:EN:PDF.

Cross, T. L., Bazron, B. J., Dennis, K. W., & Isaacs, M. R. (1989). *Towards a culturally competent system of care* (Vol. 1). Washington, DC: CASSP Technical Assistance Centre, Centre for Child Health and Mental Health Policy, Georgetown University Child Development Centre.

Daker-White, G., Beattie, A. M., Gilliard, J., & Means, R. (2002). Minority ethnic groups in dementia care: A review of service needs, service provision and models of good practice. *Aging & Mental Health, 6*(2), 101–108. http://dx.doi .org/10.1080/13607860220126835

Dana, R.H. (1998). Problems with managed mental health care for multicultural populations. *Psychological Reports, 83*(1), 283–294.

Faison, W.E., & Mintzer, J.E. (2005). The growing, ethnically diverse aging population: Is our field advancing with it? *American Journal of Geriatric Psychiatry, 13*(7), 541–544. Retrieved from http://dx.doi.org/10.1097/00019442 -200507000-00001

Gallagher-Thompson, D., Talamantes, M., Ramirez, R., & Valverde, I. (1996). Service delivery issues and recommendations for working with Mexican American family caregivers. In G. Yeo & D. Dallagher-Thompson (Eds.), *Ethnicity and the dementias* (pp. 137–152). Washington, DC: Taylor & Francis.

Guichon, J. (2007, November 27). Doctor dilemma defies easy decision. *Calgary Herald*, A14.

Guidelines on multicultural education, training, research, practice, and organizational change for psychologists. (2003) *American Psychologist, 58* (5), 377–402.

Hansen, N. D., Pepitone-Arreola-Rockwell, F., & Greene, A. F. (2000). Multicultural competence: Criteria and case examples. *Professional Psychology, Research and Practice, 31*(6), 652–660. http://dx.doi.org/10.1037/0735-7028.31.6.652

Harwood, A. (Ed.). (1981). *Ethnicity and medical care*. Cambridge, MA: Harvard University Press.

Hill, C. E. (1976). A folk medical belief system in the American South: Some practical considerations. *Southern Medical Journal, 64*, 11–17.

Ho, D. Y. F. (1995). Internalized culture, culturocentrism, and transference. *Counseling Psychologist, 23*(1), 4–24. http:// dx.doi.org/10.1177/0011000095231002

Kleinman, A. (1981). *Clients and healers in the context of culture: An exploration of the borderland between anthropology, medicine, and psychiatry*. Berkeley and Los Angeles, CA: University of California Press.

Kleinman, A., Eisenberg, L., & Good, B. (1978). Culture, illness and care: Clinical lessons from anthropological and cross-cultural research. *Annals of Internal Medicine, 88*(2), 251–258. http://dx.doi.org/10.7326/0003-4819-88-2-251

Lum, D. (1992). *Social work practice and people of color: A process-stage approach* (2nd ed.). Pacific Grove, CA: Brooks/ Cole Publishing Company.

Lynch, E. W., & Hanson, M. J. (1998). *Developing cross-cultural competence: A guide for working with children and their families*. Baltimore: Paul H. Brookes.

Martinez, R. A. (Ed.). (1978). *Hispanic culture and health care: Fact, fiction, folklore*. St Louis: CV Mosby Company.

Mason, J. (1996). *Cultural competence self-assessment questionnaire*. Portland, OR: JLM & Associates.

Mason, J. C. (1980). Ethnicity and clinical care: Indians. *Physician Assistant. Health Practitioner, 4*(11), 30–32, 39.

Muecke, M. A. (1983). Caring for Southeast Asian refugee clients in the USA. *American Journal of Public Health, 73*(4), 431–438. http://dx.doi.org/10.2105/AJPH.73.4.431

New York New Jersey Public Health Training Center (2004). *Exploring cross-cultural communication* [Course overview]. Retrieved October 22, 2014, from http://www.phtc-online.org/learning/pages/catalog/cc/default.cfm.

Opolka, J. L., Rascati, K. L., Brown, C. M., & Gibson, P. J. (2004). Ethnicity and prescription patterns for haloperidol, risperidone, and olanzapine. *Psychiatric Services (Washington, D.C.), 55*(2), 151–156. http://dx.doi.org/10.1176/appi .ps.55.2.151

Pederson, P. (1995). The culture-bound counsellor as an unintentional racist. *Canadian Journal of Counselling, 29*, 197–205.

Ridley, C. R., & Kleiner, A. J. (2003). Multicultural counselling competencies: History, themes, and issues. In D. B. Pope-Davis, H. L. K. Coleman, W. M. Liu, & R. L. Toporek (Eds.), *Handbook of multicultural competencies in counseling and psychology* (pp. 3–20). Thousand Oaks, CA: Sage. http://dx.doi.org/10.4135/9781452231693.n1

Ridley, C. R. (1995). *Overcoming unintentional racism in counseling and therapy: A practitioner's guide to intentional intervention*. Thousand Oaks, CA: Sage.

Sattar, S. P., Ahmed, M. S., Madison, J., Olsen, D. R., Bhatia, S. C., Ellahi, S., Majeed, F., Ramaswamy, S., Petty, F., Wilson, D. R. (2004). Client and physician attitudes to using medications with religiously forbidden ingredients. *Annals of Pharmacotherapy, 38*(11), 1830–1835. http://dx.doi.org/10.1345/aph.1E001

Shapiro, D. A. (1995). Finding out how psychotherapies help people change. *Psychotherapy Research, 5*(1), 1–21. http://dx.doi.org/10.1080/10503309512331331106

Snow, L. F. (1974). Folk medical beliefs and their implications for care of clients: A review based on studies among Black Americans. *Annals of Internal Medicine, 81*(1), 82–96. http://dx.doi.org/10.7326/0003-4819-81-1-82

Sue, D. W., & Sue, D. (1999). *Counseling the culturally different* (3rd ed.). New York: Wiley.

Sue, D. W. (2001). Multidimensional facets of cultural competence. *Counseling Psychologist, 29*(6), 790–821. http://dx .doi.org/10.1177/0011000001296002

Waugh, E. H., Szafran, O., & Hanafi, S. (2011). *Health Professional's Self-assessment of Cultural Competency (HPSACC) Questionnaire*. Edmonton, AB: Centre for Health and Culture. [formerly CCCSHH]

Modules and Films for Skill Development

....

Introduction to the Modules

In this section of your workbook, there are eight learning modules, one mid-course review, one end-of-course review, and one final evaluation. Modules 1 through 8 are designed to help you communicate more competently. Each module has a corresponding film (see the DVD provided at the back of this book) that helps demonstrate cultural situations that can impact clients' health care and treatment.

The reviews provide a way of evaluating your progress in cultural competency. A final evaluation is provided to help you assess your learning for the entire workbook.

Module 1: Cultural Roles in Mental Health

Film: *Depression*

LEARNING OBJECTIVES

- To be aware that culture describes both the meaning of depression and the way it is treated
- To understand that cultural roles in families play an important role in adherence to treatment
- To negotiate cultural preferences in a treatment regime

Module 2: Cultural Issues in Obtaining Consent

Film: *Informed Consent*

LEARNING OBJECTIVES

- To determine the influence of language and translation in obtaining consent
- To identify similarities and differences between the institutional culture and the client's cultural perspective(s)
- To negotiate an appropriate care solution

Module 3: Cultural Issues in Compliance

Film: *Machine That Makes Air*
LEARNING OBJECTIVES

- To perceive how community cultural roles influence personal health compliance
- To identify similarities and differences between the professional and client cultural perspective(s)
- To negotiate an appropriate, culturally sensitive care solution

Module 4: Language Diversity in Health Care

Film: *Dementia and Language Reversion*
LEARNING OBJECTIVES

- To become aware of how language diversity and language reversion influence client care
- To identify similarities and differences between the professional and client cultural perspective(s)
- To negotiate an appropriate, culturally sensitive care solution

Review of Modules 1–4: Testing Cultural Understanding

Film: *Modesty Codes and Breast Cancer*
LEARNING OBJECTIVES

- To be aware that some cultures place a religious value on the body's privacy
- To be aware that heads of families may play a key role in dealing with health issues
- To negotiate a strategy to provide care that respects perceptions of privacy

Module 5: Cultural Dimensions in Counselling

Film: *Post-Traumatic Stress*
LEARNING OBJECTIVES

- To be aware that cultural attitudes toward psychological treatment impacts effectiveness
- To negotiate about the effectiveness of counselling as the foundation for therapy
- To negotiate a commitment to PTSD treatment

Module 6: Generational Views on Personal Directives

Film: *Living Wills/Personal Directives*
LEARNING OBJECTIVES

- To be cognizant of how generational views influence medical treatment and end-of-life wishes

- To identify similarities and differences between the traditional cultural views and assimilated cultural views
- To be aware of culturally diverse views within families

Module 7: Challenging Cultural Norms

Film: *Personal Directive*
LEARNING OBJECTIVES

- To be aware of the influence of diverse religious views on end-of-life decisions
- To identify similarities and differences between the personal and institutional views on end-of-life care

Module 8: Cultural Influence in Family Decision Making

Film: *End-of-Life Issues*
LEARNING OBJECTIVES

- To understand how religious and cultural roles influence family decisions at end-of-life
- To identify similarities and differences between the professional and client cultural perspective(s)
- To negotiate an appropriate, culturally sensitive care solution

Review of Modules 5–8: Testing Cultural Understanding

Film: *Dementia and Caregiver Stress*
LEARNING OBJECTIVES

- To identify cultural influences on traditional roles in family care
- To become aware of similarities and differences between the professional and client cultural perspective(s)
- To negotiate an appropriate, culturally sensitive care plan

Final Evaluation: Cultural Issues in End-of-Life Care

Film: *No Code*
LEARNING OBJECTIVES

- To understand how ancestral and generational roles influence health care decisions
- To identify similarities and differences between the professional and client cultural perspective(s)
- To negotiate an appropriate, culturally sensitive care solution

Module 1: Cultural Roles in Mental Health

LEARNING OBJECTIVES

- To be aware that culture describes both the meaning of depression and the way it is treated
- To understand that cultural roles in families play an important role in adherence to treatment
- To negotiate cultural preferences in a treatment regime

View the film and answer the questions that follow in the workbook using the LEARN Model and BRIDGES Tool.

Film: *Depression*

This film is a case example for learning purposes only.

Synopsis of Film

Emilio is a Mexican man who is struggling with depression. He visits Dr. Damree who recommends that Emilio see a psychiatrist. Emilio's mother, Mrs. Gonzales, is very protective of her son. She reacts to the stigma associated with mental health and is concerned about what it implies for her son. Mrs. Gonzales does not want Emilio to take the medications prescribed by Dr. Damree. She sends the medications to other family members in Mexico and gives Emilio herbal medications. Resisting Dr. Damree's diagnosis, she insists that Emilio see another physician, Dr. Nguyen, who understands the cultural situation. Dr. Nguyen prescribes alternative solutions for Emilio.

Appendix F describes more details about the cultural situation related to this film and includes indications of cultural factors that can impact the client's treatment.

THINKING POINT
Cultural beliefs determine attitudes towards mental health and treatment.

Listen

Discover the Cultural Story

1. How do Emilio and his mother view Emilio's health problem? How do their viewpoints differ?

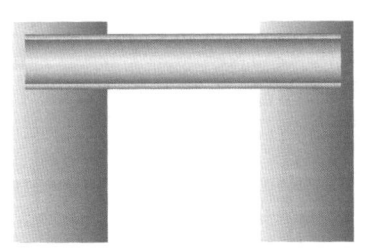

From the Film

- The role of Emilio's mother is critical.

- Alternative therapies play a role in this film.

- Relatives abroad may be a factor in adherence.

- Resistance to identifying depression as a mental health issue is important.

- Some cultures do not regard depression as a "real" illness.

2. Who is the cultural authority?

3. What information does the counselling professional not have access to regarding the use of the prescribed medication?

Explain

Explain Cultural Perspectives

1. Identify one or two of the cultural perspectives presented in this film. For instance, what do the people involved feel they must do or be?

2. Identify one or two cultural perspectives of care that are similar to or different from your own professional views.

Similarities	Differences

3. Explain your understanding of the culturally loaded words in this situation.

4. Describe how the second health professional picks up on the deeper cultural problem involved.

Acknowledge

Acknowledge the Impact of Cultural Roles on Mental Health

1. How would you tell Mrs. Gonzales you understand the cultural issues you listed on the previous page?

2. What are one or two simple things that you could do to build trust between you and this family, given the cultural views of family care in their community?

3. How does the situation in this film make sense from the mother's perspective?

4. What information is sensitive? How does that information relate to the norms, values, and beliefs of Emilio and his mother?

Recommend

Recommend Respectful and Culturally Sensitive Health Care Solutions

1. What health care solution(s) would make sense in terms of this family's issue(s)?

2. What respectful, culturally sensitive solutions would you recommend to this family? For example, what specific things do you want to include in the health care solutions that respectfully consider the client's fears?

Negotiate

Find Common Ground by Building a Competency Bridge

1. How would you discuss appropriate services to the mother and son? Think in terms of building cultural understanding between you and this family.

Counselling Plan

- Build cultural trust through understanding roles of alternative therapies.
- Improve communication with key family members/ significant others.
- Obtain better client acceptance of care plan.

L-E-A-R-N Model Summary

Cultural Roles in Mental Health

1. Summarize the cultural attitudes towards depression and mental health in this film.

2. Indicate family roles in determining counselling care.

3. Discuss ways to accommodate cultural attitudes that challenge counselling.

B-R-I-D-G-E-S Tool

Identify elements of the client's cultural perspective that will help you develop a cultural understanding.

B _____

_____

_____

R _____

_____

_____

I _____

_____

_____

D _____

_____

_____

G _____

_____

_____

E _____

_____

_____

S _____

_____

_____

Self-Reflection Exercises

For additional enrichment and further self-study, these self-reflection exercises will help your process of self-discovery, understanding, problem solving, and self-directed learning.

1. Reflect on the distinctive cultural attitudes towards mental health issues in your family and community.

2. Suggest a case you have seen where cultural attitudes required additional steps to provide counselling assistance. Describe the additional steps that were needed.

3. Indicate instances within your own cultural group where therapies are resisted because of their implications for the group.

4. What are some cultural cues you can identify?

Module 2: Cultural Issues in Obtaining Consent

LEARNING OBJECTIVES

- To determine the influence of language and translation in obtaining consent
- To identify similarities and differences between the institutional culture and the client's cultural perspective(s)
- To negotiate an appropriate care solution

View the film and answer the questions that follow in the workbook using the LEARN Model and BRIDGES Tool.

Film: *Informed Consent*

This film is a case example for learning purposes only.

Synopsis of Film

An Aboriginal diabetic woman whose leg and foot have very poor circulation has come to the hospital for surgery to increase blood circulation to her leg. She doesn't speak or read English but signed a consent form for treatment that was written in English. The significance of the consent form was apparently not properly communicated to her. The client's daughter has acted as translator and has given permission to the hospital to amputate her mother's leg, if necessary. The mother, however, wishes to walk on the path of the ancestors as a whole person and prefers to die without amputation. There is obvious conflict between what the surgeon believed he was allowed to do with the consent form and what both the daughter and her mother understood by signing the form. This film raises issues related to communication, translation, and conflicts between hospital procedure and Aboriginal beliefs.

Appendix B describes more details about the cultural situation related to this film and includes examples of cultural factors that can impact the client's health care and treatment.

THINKING POINT 
Cultural beliefs influence communication.

Listen

Discover the Cultural Story

1. What is the story in this film?

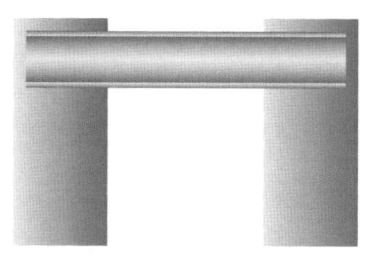

From the Film

- Elder respect is a key value in Aboriginal culture.

- Respect for personal autonomy is a highly valued principle.

- Aboriginal families prefer peer-based consultations, not an authority-based system.

- Individuals have their distinctive path to walk in this life, and others should respect that.

2. What cultural issues of obtaining consent are portrayed in the film?

Explain

Explain Cultural Perspectives

1. Identify one or two of your own cultural perspectives about obtaining consent.

2. From the film, identify one or two cultural perspectives about obtaining consent that are similar to and different from your own personal or professional views:

Similarities	Differences

3. Explain your understanding of the cultural translation problems that will most likely impact this family's care plan.

Acknowledge

Acknowledge the Impact of Language and Translation on Obtaining Consent

1. What are one or two communication issues for the daughter and her mother?

2. How would you tell the daughter that you understand the translation conflicts between hospital procedures and Aboriginal beliefs?

3. What are one or two simple things you can do to build trust, given the obvious conflict about what was communicated?

Recommend

Recommend Respectful and Appropriate Health Care Solutions

1. What health care solution(s) would make sense in terms of this family's cultural issue(s) related to obtaining consent?

2. What respectful, culturally sensitive solution(s) would you recommend for this family? For example, what specific things do you want to include in the care solution(s) that respectfully consider everyone involved?

Negotiate

Find Common Ground by Building a Competency Bridge

1. How would you build a care plan that takes this family's cultural perspective into consideration? Think in terms of building cultural understanding between you and this family.

> ### *Counselling Plan*
>
> - Build cultural understanding.
> - Improve communication.
> - Obtain better client acceptance of care plan.

2. How would you discuss your recommended care solution with this family?

L-E-A-R-N Model Summary

Cultural Issues in Obtaining Consent

1. Summarize the cultural issue(s) in obtaining consent, in terms of the mother's and daughter's cultural beliefs, values, and norms.

2. Describe an appropriate care solution for this family.

B-R-I-D-G-E-S Tool

Identify elements of the client's cultural perspective that will help you develop a cultural understanding.

B _____

_____

_____

R _____

_____

_____

I _____

_____

_____

D _____

_____

_____

G _____

_____

_____

E _____

_____

_____

S _____

_____

Self-Reflection Exercises

For additional enrichment and further self-study, these self-reflection exercises will help your process of self-discovery, understanding, problem solving, and self-directed learning.

1. Describe an experience in your personal or professional life where culture, language, or organizational procedures challenged your ability to communicate clearly.

Module 3: Cultural Issues in Compliance

LEARNING OBJECTIVES

- To perceive how community cultural roles influence personal health compliance
- To identify similarities and differences between the professional and client cultural perspective(s)
- To negotiate an appropriate, culturally sensitive care solution

View the film and answer the questions that follow in the workbook using the LEARN Model and BRIDGES Tool.

Film: *Machine That Makes Air*

This film is a case example for learning purposes only.

Synopsis of Film

The film's setting reflects the common preference among Aboriginal people for natural language and imagery of nature in everyday expression. An elderly Cree man who is the community ceremonialist and traditional healer in his Cree community has been prescribed an oxygen tank, which he calls the "machine that makes air." His wife and granddaughter (who now live in the city) have a conversation about their concerns. They are concerned about the impact that his health condition will have on his community position and responsibilities. The film depicts three problems: (a) the social roles in compliance, (b) the conflict between generations, and (c) the inner tension between loyalty to the Cree healer's ceremonial position and his own health.

Appendix B describes more details about the cultural situation related to this film and includes examples of cultural factors that can impact the client's health care and treatment.

> **THINKING POINT**
>
> The role of the client in the larger community should be part of the health care plan.

Listen

Discover the Cultural Story

1. What is the story from each individual's perspective?

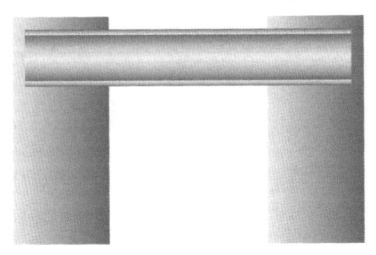

From the Film

- Aboriginal communities value specially gifted people.

- Culture plays a critical role in personal health compliance.

- Aboriginal communities give high value to group decision making.

- Adherence to Aboriginal tradition is considered more important than personal gain.

- Decision making by consensus is highly valued.

2. What are the compliance issues portrayed in the film?

Explain

Explain Cultural Perspectives

1. Identify one or two of your own cultural perspectives related to compliance.

2. From the film, identify one or two cultural perspectives related to compliance that are similar to and different from your own personal or professional views:

Similarities	Differences

3. Explain your professional understanding of the potential conflict regarding treatment compliance.

Acknowledge

Acknowledge the Impact of Community on Personal Health Compliance

1. What are one or two culturally sensitive issue(s) for the elderly Cree healer?

2. What is the community's role in the Cree healer's health?

3. What are simple things that you can do to build trust with the Cree healer and his family, given his role in the community?

Recommend

Recommend Respectful and Culturally Sensitive Health Care Solutions

1. What culturally sensitive health care solution would you suggest for the healer?

2. What are specific health care solutions that would be culturally acceptable to the healer's community?

Negotiate

Find Common Ground by Building a Competency Bridge

1. How would you discuss with the Cree healer how to build a care plan with his community role in mind? Think in terms of building cultural understanding between you and this family.

> **Counselling Plan**
>
> - Build cultural understanding.
> - Improve communication.
> - Obtain better client acceptance of care plan.

2. How would you negotiate compliance with the Cree healer?

L-E-A-R-N Model Summary

Cultural Issues in Compliance

1. Summarize the cultural issues(s) related to compliance in terms of this family's and community's cultural perspective(s).

2. Describe a culturally sensitive and appropriate care solution.

B-R-I-D-G-E-S Tool

Identify elements of the client's cultural perspective that will help you develop a cultural understanding.

B _____

_____

_____

R _____

_____

_____

I _____

_____

_____

D _____

_____

_____

G _____

_____

_____

E _____

_____

_____

S _____

_____

_____

Self-Reflection Exercises

For additional enrichment and further self-study, these self-reflection exercises will help your process of self-discovery, understanding, problem solving, and self-directed learning.

1. Reflect on a situation you were involved in wherein someone else's cultural perspectives took precedence over his or her own personal health. Describe this in terms of the communication issues portrayed in the film.

2. Describe a situation you know about wherein cultural perspectives influenced client compliance with treatment.

3. In the situations you identified, what skills can you apply that would appropriately facilitate culturally sensitive care?

. . . .

Module 4: Language Diversity in Health Care

LEARNING OBJECTIVES

- To become aware of how language diversity and language reversion influence client care
- To identify similarities and differences between the professional and client cultural perspective(s)
- To negotiate an appropriate, culturally sensitive care solution

View the film and answer the questions that follow in the workbook using the LEARN Model and BRIDGES Tool.

Film: *Dementia and Language Reversion*

This film is a case example for learning purposes only.

Synopsis of Film

A bilingual, aged woman with mixed dementia has been admitted to the hospital. As a result of mini strokes, the woman has reverted to her original French language. During the night, the woman falls and breaks her hip. The next day, at the start of a shift, a young nurse responds to a stat call and does not have the time to read the woman's chart. The nurse does not know the woman has a broken hip. She attempts to turn the woman in her bed. The aged woman screams in pain as her daughter enters the room. The daughter is upset that pain has been inflicted on her mother and contends that the nurse should have read the chart and found someone who spoke French to communicate with her mother.

Appendix C describes more details about the cultural situation related to this film and includes examples of cultural factors that can impact the client's health care and treatment.

THINKING POINT
Providing linguistically appropriate health care is an organizational and community responsibility.

Listen

Discover the Cultural Story

1. What is the story from the daughter's perspective? What concern does she have?

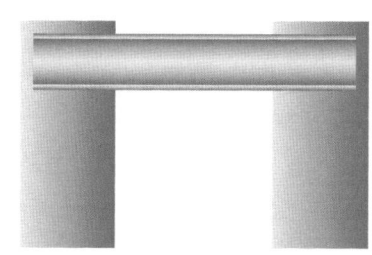

From the Film

- Francophone communities highly value the ability to communicate in the French language.

- Lack of language translation services can generate considerable controversy for a francophone community.

2. How does language play a role in the care of the patient?

Explain

Explain Cultural Perspectives

1. Comment on your professional awareness of language reversion.

2. From the film, identify one or two cultural perspectives that are similar to and different from your own personal or professional views:

Similarities	Differences

3. Provide your professional opinion of the potential health problem(s) that can arise from language issues.

Acknowledge

Acknowledge the Importance of Language Diversity in Responding to Client Care and Service

1. Why is the language issue critical for the patient and her daughter?

2. Language reversion can complicate the provision of health services. What are some implications of language reversion in counselling?

3. What are simple things that you could do to build trust with the patient and her daughter?

Recommend

Recommend Respectful and Culturally Sensitive Health Care Solutions

1. What plan would make sense in providing bilingual health care?

2. What are one or two specific things that you would include in the health care solution(s) that would respectfully consider everyone involved?

Negotiate

Find Common Ground by Building a Competency Bridge

1. How would you discuss your recommended solution with this family? Think in terms of building cultural understanding between you and this family.

> ### *Counselling Plan*
>
> - Build cultural understanding through language sensitivity.
> - Improve communication by facilitating translation.
> - Obtain better client acceptance of the counselling plan.

2. How can a translator be incorporated into the health care plan?

L-E-A-R-N Model Summary

Language Diversity in Health Care

1. Summarize the issues of language diversity in health care in terms of this family's cultural beliefs, values, and/or norms.

2. Describe a culturally sensitive and appropriate health care solution for this family.

B-R-I-D-G-E-S Tool

Identify elements of the client's cultural perspective that will help you develop a cultural understanding.

B _____

_____

_____

R _____

_____

_____

I _____

_____

_____

D _____

_____

_____

G _____

_____

_____

E _____

_____

_____

S _____

_____

Self-Reflection Exercises

For additional enrichment and further self-study, these self-reflection exercises will help your process of self-discovery, understanding, problem solving, and self-directed learning.

1. Why was bilingual care not provided for the mother?

2. Reflect on a situation in your personal or professional life where access to translation presented a challenge. Describe how that situation affects your view of language diversity.

3. Have you ever experienced a similar dilemma to the one presented in the film? Describe the situation. How did you feel? What did you learn from that experience?

4. List culturally sensitive skills you can develop to help address language diversity in health care.

Review of Modules 1–4: Testing Cultural Understanding

LEARNING OBJECTIVES

- To be aware that some cultures place a religious value on the body's privacy
- To be aware that heads of families may play a key role in dealing with health issues
- To negotiate a strategy to provide care that respects perceptions of privacy

View the film and answer the questions that follow in the workbook using the LEARN Model and BRIDGES Tool.

Film: *Modesty Codes and Breast Cancer*

This film is a case example for learning purposes only.

Synopsis of Film

Three generations of women are in a sari retail shop looking for wedding clothes: the elderly Marji, her daughter Amon, and a young Canadian woman, Mary-Beth, who is marrying Amon's son. Mary-Beth is completing her medical degree at the university. Marji is clearly in physical distress when trying on saris. Mary-Beth suggests to Amon that Marji should see a doctor because Mary-Beth suspects there is something wrong with Marji's left breast. Marji and Amon return home and have a discussion about Marji's pain. They discuss the issue of a medical examination of her breasts, and Marji's moral commitment to modesty.

Appendix E describes more details about the cultural situation and includes examples of cultural factors that can impact the client's care and treatment.

Listen

Discover the Cultural Story

1. What is the cultural story presented by Marji?

2. What is the deeper story from Marji's perspective?

3. What signs or clues did you notice that point to this deeper story?

4. Which people in this film are aware of the deeper story?

Explain

Explain Cultural Perspectives

1. Identify the cultural perspectives in this film. For instance, what do the people involved feel they must do or be?

2. Identify the cultural perspectives of care that are similar to or different from your own professional views.

3. What is your personal reaction to the perspectives of the characters in this film?

4. How do traditional cultural perspectives continue to manifest themselves?

Acknowledge

Acknowledge the Impact of Cultural Perspectives on Health Care

1. What are one or two culturally sensitive issues within this family's community?

2. How would you tell Marji that you understand the issues you listed above?

3. What are simple things that you could do to build trust between you and this family, given the cultural views of family care in this community?

4. How does the situation in this film make sense from the mother's perspective?

5. What information is sensitive? How does that information relate to the norms, values, and beliefs of the people involved?

Recommend

Recommend Respectful and Culturally Sensitive Health Care Solutions

1. What health care solution would make sense in terms of this family's cultural perspective(s) of family care?

2. What respectful, culturally sensitive solution(s) would you recommend to this family? For example, what specific things would you include in the solution(s) that respectfully consider everyone involved?

Negotiate

Find Common Ground by Building a Competency Bridge

1. How would you discuss a health care solution that takes this family's perspective into consideration? Think in terms of building a cultural understanding between you and this family.

L-E-A-R-N Model Summary

Review of Modules 1–4

1. What psychological tools/methods can be used to address the cultural issue presented in this film?

2. Describe how a professional counsellor should address this situation.

B-R-I-D-G-E-S Tool

Identify elements of the client's cultural perspective that will help you develop a cultural understanding.

B _____

_____

_____

R _____

_____

_____

I _____

_____

_____

D _____

_____

_____

G _____

_____

_____

E _____

_____

_____

S _____

_____

_____

Self-Reflection Exercises

For additional enrichment and further self-study, these self-reflection exercises will help your process of self-discovery, understanding, problem solving, and self-directed learning.

1. Describe an experience in your personal or professional life in which modesty codes influenced your client's ability to seek care.

2. What was the outcome of this situation? How could it have been handled more appropriately?

Module 5: Cultural Dimensions in Counselling

LEARNING OBJECTIVES

- To be aware that cultural attitudes toward psychological treatment impacts effectiveness
- To negotiate about the effectiveness of counselling as the foundation for therapy
- To negotiate a commitment to PTSD treatment

View the film and answer the questions that follow in the workbook using the LEARN Model and BRIDGES Tool.

Film: *Post-Traumatic Stress*

This film is a case example for learning purposes only.

Synopsis of Film

Mr. Sylvan is struggling at work from recurring nightmares about his family's fate in Cambodia. His work and happiness are suffering greatly. Dr. Brandon, the psychologist, wants Mr. Sylvan to revisit these memories to release their power. However, in Cambodia, Mr. Sylvan had been taught not to do that. In Canada, the memories torture Mr. Sylvan. During therapy, it is obvious the therapist and client share a common history of dealing with post-traumatic stress disorder (PTSD).

Appendix G describes more details about the cultural situation related to this film and includes other cultural information that can impact the client's treatment.

> THINKING POINT
>
> Cultural attitudes towards traumatic memories and how to deal with them are key elements in counselling treatments.

Listen

Discover the Cultural Story

1. How does Dr. Brandon set the stage to establish safety in the relationship with Mr. Sylvan?

2. How does Dr. Brandon open up the dialogue for a deeper, more engaging narrative with Mr. Sylvan?

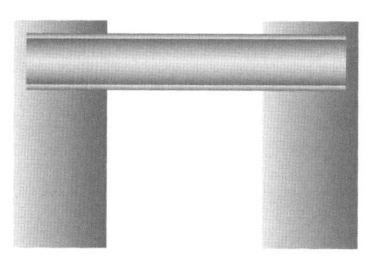

From the Film

- Attitudes toward confronting bad memories are influenced by culture.

- Roles assigned to therapy may differ from those that are foundational to psychology's traditions.

- Addressing the power of "triggers" was the strategy decided upon by this therapist.

- "Buy in" may be buttressed by the threat of job or relationship loss.

Explain

Explain Cultural Perspectives

1. Identify the process/strategies that Dr. Brandon uses to get to the root cause of Mr. Sylvan's consultation.

2. Why is Dr. Brandon focusing on the sounds to get to the narrative?

Acknowledge

Acknowledge the Impact of Cultural Perspectives on Health Care

1. How does Mr. Sylvan's cultural past impact his present situation?

2. What is gained by understanding Mr. Sylvan's cultural past?

Recommend

Recommend Respectful and Culturally Sensitive Health Care Solutions

1. How does Dr. Brandon give Mr. Sylvan another alternative to deal with his memories?

Negotiate

Find Common Ground by Building a Competency Bridge

1. How does Dr. Brandon build a care plan that takes Mr. Sylvan's cultural needs into consideration?

Counselling Plan

- Assess the effectiveness of applying the usual therapeutic model.

- Adopt a strategy that will not directly confront cultural beliefs about traumatic memory.

- Obtain client's acceptance of an indirect counselling plan.

L-E-A-R-N Model Summary

Cultural Dimensions in Counselling

1. Summarize the impact of culture on the role given to traumatic memory by the client in this film.

2. Briefly outline a culturally sensitive and appropriate counselling regime for this individual.

B-R-I-D-G-E-S Tool

Identify elements of the client's cultural perspective that will help you develop a cultural understanding.

B _____

_____

_____

R _____

_____

_____

I _____

_____

_____

D _____

_____

_____

G _____

_____

_____

E _____

_____

_____

S _____

_____

_____

Self-Reflection Exercises

For additional enrichment and further self-study, these self-reflection exercises will help your process of self-discovery, understanding, problem solving, and self-directed learning.

1. Reflect on other cases you have encountered where triggers led directly to a traumatic memory. What strategy can you use to reduce the impact of such triggers?

2. Some cultures believe there is a risk to well-being in dealing with a traumatic event directly. Does this strategy have other implications for counselling besides trauma?

3. When a client refuses to deal with deep, traumatic memories, what processes can be used to help overcome resistance?

Module 6: Generational Views on Personal Directives

LEARNING OBJECTIVES

- To be cognizant of how generational views influence medical treatment and end-of-life wishes
- To identify similarities and differences between the traditional cultural views and assimilated cultural views
- To be aware of culturally diverse views within families

View the film and answer the questions that follow in the workbook using the LEARN Model and BRIDGES Tool.

Film: *Living Wills/Personal Directives*

This film is a case example for learning purposes only.

Synopsis of Film

A Chinese woman and her son return from her brother's funeral services. Her brother's death has started the woman thinking about her own end-of-life and how she wants to be treated when she is no longer mentally competent or able to act on her own behalf. Her son is reluctant to engage in this discussion, but she insists they talk about it. She wants to have a "good death." She states that she wants to have a written personal directive to convey her desire for "no heroics" in an end-of-life situation. She wants to "go peacefully." Because he is the eldest son, she wants him to be her personal agent. The son agrees to comply with his mother's wishes as a way of honouring her.

Appendix D described more details about the cultural situation related to this film and includes examples of cultural factors that can impact the client's health care and treatment.

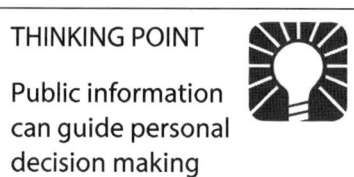

THINKING POINT

Public information can guide personal decision making

Listen

Discover the Cultural Story

1. What is the story from each individual's perspective in this film?

2. What are the generational views portrayed in the film?

Explain

Explain Cultural Perspectives

1. Identify one or two of your own perspectives on personal directives.

2. Identify one or two perspectives of personal directives or end-of-life wishes presented in the film that are similar to and different from your own personal or professional views:

Similarities	Differences

3. How would you explain to the son your understanding of the cultural problem(s) that will most likely impact this family's decision making?

Acknowledge

Acknowledge the Generational Gap in Fulfilling End-of-Life Wishes

1. What are the culturally sensitive issues for the woman and her son?

2. Why do you think the son is culturally reluctant to fulfill his mother's wishes for end-of-life medical treatment?

Recommend

Recommend Respectful and Culturally Sensitive Health Care Solutions

1. What respectful, culturally sensitive assistance would you offer to the son? For example, what are specific things that you would want to include in counselling him?

2. What value would personal directives have for this multigenerational family?

Negotiate

Find Common Ground by Building a Competency Bridge

1. How could you provide assistance so that a personal directive could accommodate both the woman's and the son's cultural perspectives?

> **Counselling Plan**
> - Improve communication by accepting the role superiority of the elder.
> - Obtain better client acceptance of the care plan by asking if it is culturally compliant.

2. What would your recommended solution(s) be for this family?

L-E-A-R-N Model Summary

Generational Views on Personal Directives

1. Summarize the generational views on personal directives in terms of this family's cultural beliefs, values, and norms.

2. Briefly describe a culturally sensitive and appropriate counselling strategy for this family.

B-R-I-D-G-E-S Tool

Identify elements of the client's cultural perspective that will help you develop a cultural understanding.

B _____

_____

_____

R _____

_____

_____

I _____

_____

_____

D _____

_____

_____

G _____

_____

_____

E _____

_____

_____

S _____

_____

_____

Self-Reflection Exercises

For additional enrichment and further self-study, these self-reflection exercises will help your process of self-discovery, understanding, problem solving, and self-directed learning.

1. Describe a situation in your professional life where personal directives or end-of-life wishes challenged traditional roles of family care.

2. What is the attitude toward personal directives in your culture?

3. Describe one or two traditional cultural views regarding dying.

Module 7: Challenging Cultural Norms

LEARNING OBJECTIVES

- To be aware of the influence of diverse religious views on end-of-life decisions
- To identify similarities and differences between the personal and institutional views on end-of-life care

View the film and answer the questions that follow in the workbook using the LEARN Model and BRIDGES Tool.

Film: *Personal Directive*

This film is a case example for learning purposes only.

Synopsis of Film

A sorrowful woman is met by her daughter in the waiting room of the hospital where the woman just witnessed the death of her brother. She is concerned not only with his death but also the manner of his dying on life-support equipment and evident conflict within his family. His children did not know what his wishes were for his end-of-life. The woman makes the case that the francophone elderly in her region have solid faith and do not want to delay their earthly life unduly, especially when life-support procedures have no effective outcome. She conveys to her daughter that she wants to define the way she herself will be treated at the end of her life through the use of a personal directive, signed by a lawyer, so she does not face the same situation as her brother. She wants "no fancy medical stuff" and wishes to "go as God wills it."

Appendix C describes more details about the cultural situation related to this film and includes examples of cultural factors that can impact the client's health care and treatment.

THINKING POINT
Individuals within cultural communities may have differing norms, values, and beliefs.

Listen

Discover the Cultural Story

1. What is the story in this film?

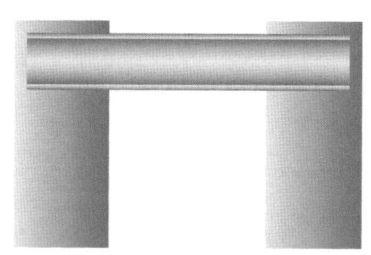

From the Film

- Religious values may play a key role in end-of-life decision making.

- Attitudes toward personal directives may vary among and within different cultural groups.

- Religious and cultural views may vary between generations.

2. What are the cultural norms portrayed in the film?

Explain

Explain Religious Perspectives

1. Identify one or two of your own religious or cultural perspectives related to end-of-life care.

2. From the film, identify one or two cultural perspectives related to end-of-life care that are similar to and different from your own personal or professional views:

Similarities	*Differences*

3. Explain your understanding of the cultural problem(s) that will most likely impact this family's end-of-life care decisions.

Acknowledge

Acknowledge the Impact of Religious Perspectives on Hospital Protocol and End-of-Life Directives

1. What are the culturally sensitive issue(s) for the woman and her daughter?

2. What are simple things that you could do to build a trusting relationship with this family?

Recommend

Recommend Respectful and Culturally Sensitive Health Care Solutions

1. What health care solution(s) would make sense in terms of this family's religious perspectives?

2. What respectful, culturally sensitive solution(s) would you recommend to the daughter? For example, what are one or two specific things that you would include in the care solution(s) so that end-of-life care would work for everyone involved?

Negotiate

Find Common Ground by Building a Competency Bridge

1. How would you build a solution that takes the mother's religious perspective into consideration? Think in terms of building cultural understanding between this family and professional protocols.

Counselling Plan

- Build cultural understanding into relationships with ethnically distinctive clients.

- Improve communication with language sensitivity.

- Obtain better client acceptance of the care plan by making sure it addresses cultural dimensions.

2. How would you discuss your recommended solution with this family?

L-E-A-R-N Model Summary

Challenging Cultural Norms

1. Summarize the cultural challenge(s) in terms of this family's cultural and religious beliefs, values, and norms.

2. Briefly describe an appropriate counselling strategy for this family.

B-R-I-D-G-E-S Tool

Identify elements of the client's cultural perspective that will help you develop a cultural understanding.

B _____

_____

_____

R _____

_____

_____

I _____

_____

_____

D _____

_____

_____

G _____

_____

_____

E _____

_____

_____

S _____

_____

_____

Self-Reflection Exercises

For additional enrichment and further self-study, these self-reflection exercises will help your process of self-discovery, understanding, problem solving, and self-directed learning.

1. Both the woman and her daughter are at different life stages. How would you describe the generational difference between the mother and daughter?

2. Professionals deal with people as individuals, but those individuals are also part of larger families. In what ways might family decisions affect professional protocols and professional care?

3. How would you approach, in a sensitive and respectful way, the family and client in terms of their end-of-life wishes? How would you assist a family signing a personal directive?

Module 8: Cultural Influence in Family Decision Making

LEARNING OBJECTIVES

- To understand how religious and cultural roles influence family decisions at end-of-life
- To identify similarities and differences between the professional and client cultural perspective(s)
- To negotiate an appropriate, culturally sensitive care solution

View the film and answer the questions that follow in the workbook using the LEARN Model and BRIDGES Tool.

Film: *End-of-Life Issues*

This film is a case example for learning purposes only.

Synopsis of Film

A Muslim father had a severe heart attack and was without oxygen for thirty minutes. The doctors have determined that there is no brain activity. His son and daughter are trying to decide what to do. They need to decide whether or not to disconnect him from life support. To their knowledge, their father did not have a personal directive. The critical issue is whether or not there is hope of him recovering, as the tenets of Islam are not to interfere with end-of-life. They decide to let him go peacefully. He will be transferred to a palliative care unit where he will receive compassionate care, comfort, and symptom management in the last phase of his life. The services of an Imam from the mosque will also be available there.

Appendix A describes more details about the cultural situation related to this film and includes examples of cultural factors that can impact the client's health care and treatment.

THINKING POINT

Culturally competent care involves community partnerships.

Listen

Discover the Cultural Story

1. What is the story in this film?

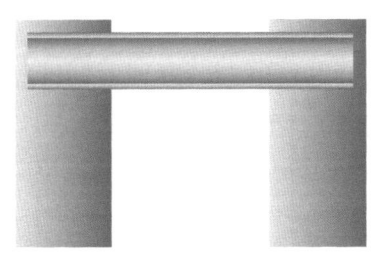

From the Film

- Decisions at the critical moments of Islamic end-of-life are left to the family.

- Prolonging life artificially is regarded as unacceptable in Islamic belief.

- If there is no brain activity, God is presumed to have taken the individual believer.

2. What is the family decision-making issue portrayed in the film?

- Authority to speak for the family normally resides with the eldest male.

- Eldest males need to arrange for an alternate support system for their families.

Explain

Explain Decision-Making Perspectives

1. Does your own family have decision-making perspectives related to compassionate care?

2. From the film, identify one or two cultural decision-making processes that are similar to and different from your own personal and professional views:

Similarities	Differences

3. How would you explain to the son and daughter your understanding of the cultural problem(s) that will most likely impact this family's decision making about end-of-life care for the father?

Acknowledge

Acknowledge the Impact of Family Decision Making on Palliative Care

1. What are the culturally sensitive issues for the young people?

2. What are some simple things you could do to build a trusting relationship with the family?

Recommend

Recommend Respectful and Culturally Sensitive Health Care Solutions

1. What health care solution(s) would make sense in terms of this family's decision-making perspectives?

2. What respectful, culturally sensitive care solution(s) would you recommend to the young people that respectfully consider everyone involved?

Negotiate

Find Common Ground by Building a Competency Bridge

1. How would you build a solution that takes the children's cultural family decision making into consideration? Think of a solution in terms of building cultural understanding between you and this family.

> ### *Counselling Plan*
>
> - Build cultural understanding with awareness of distinctive Muslim teachings about elders.
> - Improve communication by identifying points of religious difference.
> - Obtain better client acceptance of the counselling plan by verbally acknowledging distinctive cultural viewpoints.

2. How would you discuss your recommended care solution with this family?

L-E-A-R-N Model Summary

Cultural Influences in Family Decision Making

1. Summarize the cultural influence in family decision-making role(s) in terms of this family's cultural beliefs, values, and norms.

2. Briefly describe a culturally sensitive and appropriate care plan for this family.

B-R-I-D-G-E-S Tool

Identify elements of the client's cultural perspective that will help you develop a cultural understanding.

B _____

_____

_____

R _____

_____

_____

I _____

_____

_____

D _____

_____

_____

G _____

_____

_____

E _____

_____

_____

S _____

_____

_____

Self-Reflection Exercises

For additional enrichment and further self-study, these self-reflection exercises will help your process of self-discovery, understanding, problem solving, and self-directed learning.

1. One of the important issues for the young people in this film is the timing of death. Reflect upon different perspectives about when death occurs.

2. This film portrays health care professionals working together as team. How did the team assist the children?

3. What are the professional skills you could develop in order to be a client advocate?

Review of Modules 5–8: Testing Cultural Understanding

LEARNING OBJECTIVES

- To identify cultural influences on traditional roles in family care
- To become aware of similarities and differences between the professional and client cultural perspective(s)
- To negotiate an appropriate, culturally sensitive care plan

View the film and answer the questions that follow in the workbook, using the LEARN Model and BRIDGES Tool.

Film: *Dementia and Caregiver Stress*

This film is a case example for learning purposes only.

Synopsis of Film

A young Muslim daughter, Nadia, is caring for her widowed father who has Alzheimer's disease. The father does not recognize his daughter anymore. He wanders away from home and needs constant care. As an unwed daughter, Nadia feels a religious-sanctioned responsibility to care for her father. However, the care is a burden on her. She cannot sleep, does not go out socially except to the mosque, and is physically and psychologically stressed. Nadia's friend is very concerned about Nadia's health. The friend learns that Nadia is the primary caregiver and has very few supports in place to help her through this difficult time.

Appendix A describes more details about the cultural situation related to this film and includes examples of cultural factors that can impact the client's health care and treatment.

Listen

Discover the Cultural Story

1. What is the story in this film?

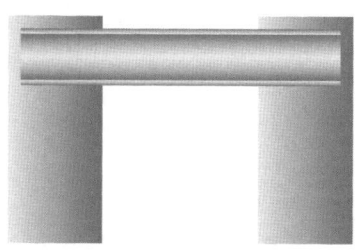

From the Film

- Nurturing roles are usually assigned to women by the family and community.

- It is the family's responsibility to take care of the elderly.

- There is reluctance to ask for community assistance because of the family's religious responsibility.

2. What are the traditional roles of family care portrayed in the film?

- Authority to speak for the family normally resides with the eldest male.

- Eldest males need to arrange for an alternate support system.

Explain

Explain Cultural Perspectives

1. Identify one or two of your own cultural perspectives of family care.

2. From the film, identify one or two cultural perspectives of care that are similar to and different from your own personal and professional views:

Similarities	Differences

3. Explain your understanding of the cultural problem(s) that will most likely impact caregiving in the family.

Acknowledge

Acknowledge the Impact of Cultural Perspectives on Traditional Family Care

1. What are one or two culturally sensitive issue(s) within this family's community?

2. How would you tell Nadia that you understand the issues you listed above?

3. What are simple things that you could do to build trust between you and this family, given their traditional views of family care?

Recommend

Recommend Respectful and Culturally Sensitive Health Care Solutions

1. What counselling solution(s) would make sense in terms of this family's cultural perspective(s) of family care?

2. What culturally sensitive solution(s) would you recommend to this family that respectfully consider everyone involved?

Negotiate

Find Common Ground by Building a Competency Bridge

1. Build a care plan that takes this family's cultural perspective into consideration. Think in terms of building cultural understanding between you and this family.

> ### *Counselling Plan*
>
> - Build cultural understanding.
> - Improve communication.
> - Obtain better client acceptance of the care plan.

2. How would you discuss your recommended care solution with this family?

L-E-A-R-N Model Summary

Traditional Roles of Family Care

1. Summarize the traditional care role(s) in terms of this family's cultural beliefs, values, and norms.

2. Describe a culturally sensitive and appropriate care plan for this family.

B-R-I-D-G-E-S Tool

Identify elements of the client's cultural perspective that will help you develop a cultural understanding.

B _____

_____

_____

R _____

_____

_____

I _____

_____

_____

D _____

_____

_____

G _____

_____

_____

E _____

_____

_____

S _____

_____

Self-Reflection Exercises

For additional enrichment and further self-study, these self-reflection exercises will help your process of self-discovery, understanding, problem solving, and self-directed learning.

1. Reflect on an experience in your personal or professional life where someone else's traditional perspectives of care challenged your own. Describe this experience in terms of conflicting beliefs, values, or norms.

2. Describe a situation where you helped someone better understand how things work in a particular culture that is not his or her own, or describe a situation where someone else did that for you.

Final Evaluation: Cultural Issues in End-of-Life Care

LEARNING OBJECTIVES

- To understand how ancestral and generational roles influence health care decisions
- To identify similarities and differences between the professional and client cultural perspective(s)
- To negotiate an appropriate, culturally sensitive care solution

View the film and answer the questions that follow in the workbook using the LEARN Model and BRIDGES Tool.

Film: *No Code*

This film is a case example for learning purposes only.

Synopsis of Film

An elderly Chinese man is in declining health due to aspiration pneumonia attributed to multiple strokes. He is not responding to all the available medical treatment modalities and now needs total care. The female physician on duty discusses the situation with his three children. Her professional advice is that he be sent to a palliative care unit where he will receive compassionate care and comfort as he approaches death peacefully. She explains that compassionate care implies "no code" (no resuscitation). This discussion results in tension and conflict between the client's children and physician. The children are upset because they see sending their father to a palliative care facility like "giving up." They stress that it is their "duty as good children" to provide the best possible care for their father. They cannot agree to "no code."

Appendix D describes more details about the cultural situation related to this film and includes examples of cultural factors that can impact the client's health care and treatment.

Listen

Discover the Cultural Story

1. What is the story in this film?

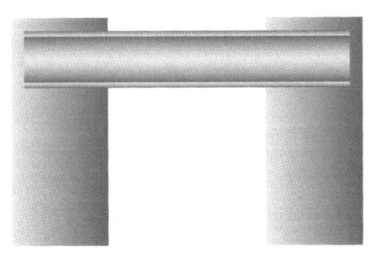

From the Film

- Chinese culture has been significantly impacted by Confucian values.

- Personal identity involves a strong ancestral component.

- In the family, ultimate decision making rests with the eldest son or the oldest or most respected family member, who can be female.

2. What are the ancestral roles in acute care portrayed in the film?

Explain

Explain Cultural Perspectives

1. Identify one or two of your own cultural perspectives related to end-of-life care.

2. From the film, identify one or two cultural perspectives of care that are similar to and different from your own personal and professional views:

Similarities	Differences

3. Explain your understanding of the cultural problem(s) that will most likely impact this family's care plan.

Acknowledge

Acknowledge the Influence of Cultural Perspectives in End-of-Life Care

1. What are the culturally sensitive issues for the children?

2. How would you tell the children that you understand their concern for maintaining ancestral respect? How do their concerns differ from the goals of palliative care?

3. What are one or two simple things that you could do to build a trusting relationship with the family?

Recommend

Recommend Respectful and Culturally Sensitive Health Care Solutions

1. What health care solution(s) would make sense in terms of this family's cultural perspective(s) of palliative care?

2. What respectful, culturally sensitive solution(s) would you recommend to the young people that respectfully consider everyone involved?

Negotiate

Find Common Ground by Building a Competency Bridge

1. How would you build a care plan that takes the children's cultural perspective into consideration? Think in terms of building cultural understanding between you and this family.

Counselling Plan
• Build on Chinese cultural understanding.
• Improve communication by determining the primary caregiver.
• Obtain better client acceptance of the care plan through sensitivity to status.

2. How would you discuss your recommended care solution(s) with the children?

L-E-A-R-N Model Summary

Cultural Differences in End-of-Life Care

1. Summarize the conflicts between this family's beliefs, norms, and values and the culture of palliative care.

2. Describe a culturally sensitive and appropriate care solution for this family.

B-R-I-D-G-E-S Tool

Identify elements of the client's cultural perspective that will help you develop a cultural understanding.

B _____

_____

_____

R _____

_____

_____

I _____

_____

_____

D _____

_____

_____

G _____

_____

_____

E _____

_____

_____

S _____

_____

_____

Self-Reflection Exercises

For additional enrichment and further self-study, these self-reflection exercises will help your process of self-discovery, understanding, problem solving, and self-directed learning.

1. How would you respond if you were in a professional situation where there was a conflict between institutional norms and the client's cultural norms?

2. The film portrays a rigid impasse. The physician raised the "no code" issue with the children. The children responded with rejection. Is there a way to mediate the rigidity that you see in the film? What mediation skills could you develop to negotiate this impasse?

3. What are the negative, non-verbal dimensions in this film that need to be discussed? If you were there, what would you say to help the children in their decision? What would you say to the physician?

Evaluating Cultural Competence

Congratulations! You've Finished the Workbook

Go back to the introduction and retake the HPSACC Questionnaire (Psychology Version). Compare your responses from the first self-assessment with your responses to the second self-assessment. This will give you a snapshot of areas of improvement. Your responses will also indicate how you can continue to improve your cultural competence during your professional career.

Study Notes

Please feel free to write your study notes on this page.

Appendices

Appendices A through G include information to help you answer the questions in the modules, reviews, and final evaluation.

Key to Appendices

Appendix	Module or Review	Cultural Perspective	LEARN Model and Helpful Hints for:	Page
Appendix A	Module 8	Muslim	Cultural Influence in Family Decision Making	133
	Review of Modules 5–8	Muslim	Traditional Roles of Family Care	137
Appendix B	Module 2	Aboriginal	Cultural Issues in Obtaining Consent	144
	Module 3	Aboriginal	Cultural Issues in Compliance	148
Appendix C	Module 4	Francophone	Language Diversity in Health Care	156
	Module 7	Francophone	Challenging Cultural Norms	159
Appendix D	Module 6	Chinese	Generational Views on Personal Directives	167
	Final Evaluation	Chinese	Cultural Issues in End-of-Life Care	171
Appendix E	Review of Modules 1–4	Sikh	Modesty Codes and Breast Cancer	177
Appendix F	Module 1	Hispanic	Cultural Roles in Mental Health/Depression	183
Appendix G	Module 5	Southeast Asian/ Cambodian	Cultural Dimensions in Counselling/Post-Traumatic Stress	190

Appendix A

Muslim Cultural Perspectives

1. Muslim Protocols of Interaction

  a. Professional relations can have a gendered dimension. That is, male health care providers may be viewed with more respect than females.

  b. Generally speaking, two unrelated people should not be alone if one is male and the other female. For example, a female homecare nurse can help with getting a male client ready for a bath, but she should not physically touch/bathe the male client. The bathing is done by his wife or a male relative. In a hospital/institution situation, this should be negotiated.

  c. There is universal reluctance to disrobe (sustained modesty code adherence).

  d. Females will be more reluctant to discuss sexual issues and/or have an obstetrical or breast examination with a male physician than they would with a female physician.

  e. Female clients may be uncomfortable with male nurses.

  f. Some female clients may be reluctant to make eye contact with a male physician. It is generally understood that Muslim women will not look an unrelated male in the eye.

  g. In some conservative Muslim communities, it is not acceptable for a physician to shake a client's hand if that client is of the opposite gender.

  h. Authority to speak for the family normally resides with the eldest male of the immediate family, or the nearest and eldest male relative.

  i. Nurturing roles are usually assigned to women.

  j. After touching a dog, a person must wash his or her hands before touching a person.

2. Muslim Language and Communication

  a. There is a trend to ask male family members (son, older brother) to translate in a public situation.

  b. Elders prefer to be communicated with in their first language for better understanding. Language differences play a larger role among the elderly due to limited command of the English language.

  c. Joking is taboo between psychologist and client, until the professional relationship develops into well-known acquaintance.

3. Provision of Health Care by Community and Organizations

  a. There is a reluctance to have medical history discussed openly with the client and family. Family members may be concerned about how medical information may affect the client's mental attitude.

b. Some families may follow Islamic Law, wherein the nearest male relative inherits the responsibility for the family wealth and is critical for family continuity. For example, a younger male child with three older female siblings will be responsible for the family wealth.

4. **Decision Making and Caregiving**

a. According to the traditional view of the Qur'an's message, it is the family's responsibility to take care of the elderly. Secular institutionalization is not regarded as an acceptable alternative, unless the individual must have continuous professional care.

b. There is a cultural tendency for the first son's wife or the youngest unmarried daughter to be responsible for caregiving.

c. Although care of the elderly is the family's responsibility, family members may ask the community for help if needed.

5. **Muslim Beliefs, Values, and Health Care Outcome Expectations**

a. It is important to communicate with the most influential and oldest male when concerning a male or female client. A man's wife is consulted when it comes to decision making about him.

6. **Unique Muslim End-of-Life Issues**

a. Bedside attendance is usually maintained for the dying, and all assistance should be provided to the family so they can spend the last moments in privacy.

b. Life and death is "in the hands of Allah." Until end-of-life, the community will desire everything medically possible for clients, including medical intervention and food and water. However, the introduction of artificial life systems poses a problem since believers do not wish to interfere with the will of God concerning death.

c. If an individual's brain indicates lack of activity, God is presumed to have taken the believer. Prolonging life artificially is unacceptable in Islamic belief.

d. Decisions at the critical moment of end-of-life are left to the family.

e. Death rites include washing of the body and same-day burial in a shroud. The most important rite is the final prayer with members of the community in the mosque. Interment is on one side, with the face pointing toward Mecca.

Module 8: Cultural Influence in Family Decision Making (LEARN Model)

Listen *respectfully to the client's perception of the problem. Get the cultural story.*

Listen to the son's perspective that end-of-life is deemed to be in the hands of God and that no extraordinary attempt should be made to keep an individual alive when it is his or her time to be called.

Explain *your understanding of this family's cultural perceptions.*

Explain to the son and daughter that there is no brain activity and it is highly unlikely that their father will recover. There is no available curative treatment, so palliative care is the only option at the last phase of life.

Acknowledge *the impact of cultural perspectives on traditional roles of family care.*

Acknowledge that end-of-life issues for Muslims are extremely stressful because of the need to mediate between the belief that all life is in God's hands and the procedures established by the health care system when someone is very ill. Acknowledge that for Muslims, determining the point at which end-of-life occurs is the key to family decision making.

Recommend *a culturally sensitive health care solution.*

Recommend that psychologists should assist in determining the point when end-of-life has occurred and recognize this issue as critical to Muslim believers.

Negotiate *common ground that builds a competency bridge.*

Negotiate with the family (usually the oldest son) about a common understanding of when death has occurred.

Module 8: Helpful Hints for Culturally Sensitive Care Plan Solutions that Consider Family Decision Making

1. What is the son's role in the decision-making process?

Discussion points:

- Traditional Muslim families stress the public decision-making role of male household members. The young man's attempt to decide what to do is based on the traditional view that he has to effect the decision.

2. What is the son trying to determine?

Discussion points:

- Traditionally, Sunni Muslims regard the moment of death to be in the hands of God. When it is time, the individual is deemed to be called by the Angel of Death, who takes the soul to the other world. Excessive medical intervention can be regarded as a human attempt to interfere with God's will for a person's life. Still, it is only when life is no longer viable that one can disconnect the machines. That "moment" is the problem the brother and sister are wrestling with.

3. How did the doctor's communication with the son help or hinder the son's understanding of the situation?

Discussion points:

- From the perspective of the family, there was too much medical jargon in the discussion. Their only concern was whether they had to regard their father as already called by the Angel of Death.

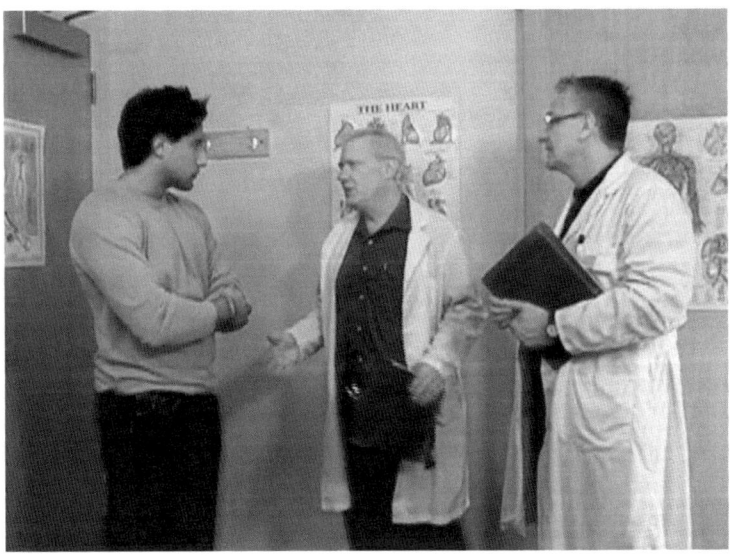

4. Who could help with the decision-making process if the eldest son were not available?

Discussion points:

- In this community, the next available male family member and peer of the client (brother or uncle) can help with decision making.

- It would not be wise to continue discussions unless another male member of the family is called to assist. Certainly, the women in the family could offer their points of view, but it would be culturally sensitive not to press the issue with them but and instead ask them to bring in the senior member of their family.

5. What is the Muslim group's belief about end-of-life? How is this at odds with hospital protocol?

Discussion points:

- Muslim belief about end-of-life is that human intervention should not prolong a vegetative state of life. Upon death, the person's face should be turned to Mecca.

- Without clear guidance, as is provided by a proper personal directive, hospital procedure requires the client be kept on a respirator.

Module 8: Cultural Understanding (BRIDGES Tool)

Insight into the values, beliefs, and attitudes of clients brings a deeper awareness of their cultural perspectives. BRIDGES helps us gain deeper cultural understanding.

Beliefs, Values, Norms: An understanding of Muslim end-of-life beliefs will assist greatly in helping these young people. They must decide whether the Angel of Death has indeed taken the soul of their father. Once that decision is made, they will be able to address the rest of his care.

Roles and Relationships with Family/Relatives: In this situation, the young man realizes he must make a decision on behalf of the family, so he must know exactly what has occurred. His role as head of the family becomes dominant.

Identify Language, Literacy, Communication: Communication, language, and even standard Muslim phrases demonstrate that religious values must take precedence at this moment. Muslim values indicate that humans should not interfere with someone who has departed to be with God.

Decision Making Methods/Practices: The family must make a decision so they can inform community members and plan end-of-life visitations and funeral rites.

Group, Community, Organizations: In a traditional society, paying respects to the departed is a community requirement. That is why ascertaining the exact nature of the father's condition is essential.

Extraordinary Issues in Health (end-of-life, childbirth, etc.): Several cultural and religious acts must be undertaken at the end of someone's life, and the community's perception of the family members' activities at death will contribute to the perception of how "good" the family is. It is a critical time for everyone.

Share Understanding of Cultures, Reach Common Ground, and Compromise: Most religious communities place emphasis on the passing of a loved one, so counselling professionals will encounter different models of what should be done at end-of-life. Being aware of the stressful issues and assisting in a smooth transition will provide a common ground for meeting the family's needs.

Review of Modules 5–8: Traditional Roles of Family Care (LEARN Model)

Listen *respectfully to the client's perception of the problem. Get the cultural story.*

Listen as the daughter willingly accepts her religious-sanctioned responsibility to care for her father. Qur'anic doctrine assigns responsibility for a family senior's well-being directly to family members. An unwed daughter or eldest son's wife is assigned the caregiver role. Professional or community support is regarded with skepticism because it is not supported by the Muslim scripture.

Explain *your understanding of the family's cultural perceptions.*

Explain to the daughter that she has become a stressed caregiver who needs help herself. The caregiving demands of her ailing father have become too much for her to handle alone.

Acknowledge *the impact of cultural perspectives related to traditional roles of family care.*

Acknowledge the daughter's commitment to the Muslim doctrine. Agree with the Qur'an's assignment of caregiving responsibility. Support the daughter in her commitment to her father. Note that this implies an extended-family context that may not be available to her in Canada. You may wish to undergo community-awareness training to help support the daughter's commitment to her father.

Recommend *a culturally sensitive health care solution.*

Recommend that the family engage a Muslim caregiving team so that adequate respite is given to the caregiver daughter. Suggest that the cultural community learn more about the severity of the problem and provide direct support to the daughter. Discuss more than one way of handling the situation so that the doctrine remains intact.

Negotiate *common ground that builds a competency bridge.*

Negotiate with the daughter so that she seeks assistance in the face of her depressed state. Negotiate with Muslim community members to provide the familial support assumed in the Qur'anic injunction but obviously not available in the town.

Review of Modules 5–8: Helpful Hints for Culturally Sensitive Care Plan Solutions that Consider Traditional Family Care

1. Why does the daughter feel that she cannot ask for help?

Discussion points:

- She and her community hold that this is her responsibility, given by God according to Qur'anic prescription. As a devout believer, she does not wish to shirk her duty.

2. Why has the daughter not accessed health care and community support?

Discussion points:

- Going outside her family for assistance is an action that she is not able to accept because of her position in the family and the implications for her religious duty.

3. What can the doctor do to help with this situation?

Discussion points:

- When she comes to the office with her father, it would be wise for the doctor or counselling professional to discuss her situation and suggest some way of helping her cope. Perhaps a professional's insistence might motivate her to appeal directly to other community members, especially if the counselling professional offers to train them or help them find training.

4. What is the daughter's understanding of her father's disease?

Discussion points:

- She has only rudimentary knowledge of her father's condition and does not know the significance of her father's behaviour sometimes, as expressed in her need to hide the knives without acknowledging the danger.
- She appears to have very limited understanding of medical knowledge about the progress of dementias.

5. Caregiver burnout is a common problem among caregivers. How could Muslim community leaders address this issue?

Discussion points:

- The eldest brother needs to contact community leaders to arrange for an alternate support system.
- The daughter needs regular respite if she is to continue as caregiver.

Review of Modules 5–8: Cultural Understanding (BRIDGES Tool)

Insight into the values, beliefs, and attitudes of clients brings a deeper awareness of their cultural perspectives. BRIDGES helps us gain deeper cultural understanding.

Beliefs, Values, Norms: Awareness of the stress some religious cultures place on caring for elders as a mark of a righteous person/family will aid in understanding why the daughter did not feel she could or should seek outside help. Some older members of some communities regard dementia as a kind of disease that has status implications in the community.

Roles and Relationships with Family/Relatives: In this community, and for this daughter, the daughter's true responsibility is caring for her father, regardless of how problematic that is.

Identify Language, Literacy, Communication: Issues raised with regard to who cares for elders often has cultural implications; sometimes cultural meaning blends with religious beliefs. Her family identifies with a distinctive conception, found in many conservative cultures, that women are always the primary caregivers, so communications centred on that perception hold sway over her entire life.

Decision Making Methods/Practices: Any attempt to convey how difficult the task might be may be interpreted by some community members as weakness, or lack of ability, so most of the crucial decisions seem beyond her control.

Group, Community, Organizations: The environment into which the Qur'an was given was a closely knit, complex, tribal network, with many hands to help with the elderly. This small community does not have the resources of Meccan society, and the group has to decide how best to handle this fact. A sensitive counselling professional might aid in finding resources to help the daughter in a way that will not undercut her position and role.

Extraordinary Issues in Health (end-of-life, childbirth, etc.): End-of-life care brings many different perspectives; the care of the elderly can be a divisive issue in some communities. It may be stressful for women members who are expected to be caregivers.

Share Understanding of Cultures, Reach Common Ground, and Compromise: An awareness of the stress brought on by these matters will allow the health care provider to find common ground with the community and the daughter. It obviously assists the community when the health care provider is aware of its norms, beliefs, and values.

RESOURCE MATERIALS

Aswad, B. C. (1991). Yemeni and Lebanese Muslim immigrant women in Southeast Dearborn Michigan. In E. H. Waugh, S. M. Abu-Laban, & R. B. Qureshi (Eds.), *Muslim families in North America* (pp. 256–281). Edmonton, AB: University of Alberta Press.

Lawrence, P., & Rozmus, C. (2001). Culturally sensitive care of the Muslim client. *Journal of Transcultural Nursing, 12*(3), 228–233. http://dx.doi.org/10.1177/104365960101200307

Sachedina, A. (2009, June 12). Right to die?: Muslim views about end of life decisions. Retrieved from http://people .virginia.edu/~aas/article/article3.htm

Waugh, E. H. (1999). *The Islamic tradition: Religious beliefs and healthcare decisions.* Chicago: The Park Ridge Center.

Appendix B

Aboriginal Cultural Perspectives

1. **Aboriginal Protocols of Interaction**

   a. There is limited eye contact, shaking of hands, or male–female interaction. For example, a mother-in-law does not directly address her son-in-law, and a father-in law does not directly address his daughter-in-law. Communication is conducted via the daughter or son, respectively.

   b. History of present illness is often best obtained through stories or narratives and not by direct questioning regarding body functions. Oral tradition influences the manner of exchanging dialogue.

   c. It is believed that a life-limiting prognosis is not under the authority of the physician or health care professionals but is dealt with in the realm of the spirit world (e.g., traditional healer or peers in a talking circle).

   d. A formal, structured, health care encounter may not provide the best interaction. Talking circles consisting of peers are very beneficial in developing relationships and conveying information about diagnoses. The best evidence indicates that standardized tests should be avoided.

   e. Communal values play a significant role in personal life decisions.

2. **Aboriginal Language and Communication**

   a. Aboriginal language may not have equivalent terms to describe some diseases (e.g., dementia). Dementia may be identified by symptoms such as forgetfulness and inattentiveness. This implies that some health issues may be regarded as simply a stage in one's age-evolution.

   b. Communication style is also distinctive. Trust time is required—one needs to provide refreshments and to develop an atmosphere of friendship and casualness to gain trust. At times, silence is also considered good communication. In the old days, smoking together was a sign of mutual sharing and responsiveness. First encounters might best be more social than medical, and histories might better be left until after trust has been built.

   c. Some clients may not answer personal queries because of respect for their family or because they are sensitive to power differentials with the health care providers. They may also defer to a family member or a person of authority in their culture.

   d. Asserting who translates information (e.g., family vs. professional) can generate miscommunication and conflict. Family translators may be preferred so that sensitive information is kept within the family circle. This also provides the family more control over the situation.

e. Elderly Aboriginal clients, especially when they are ill, prefer their original language as the mode of communication. Care should be taken in the translation of critical information, such as likely outcomes.

3. **Provision of Health Care by Community and Organizations**

a. Respect for personal independence and autonomy is a highly valued principle among Aboriginal people. Non-intervention and respect shown by the nuclear family is the rule. There is limited extended family involvement, unless they have been close in their personal relationships, and then only when it is apparent that the individual needs help.

b. Due to a general decline in nuclear family units, it is important to monitor the needs of elderly Aboriginal clients, as responsibility may have shifted from the nuclear family to the community. In many cases, a spokesperson will emerge during consultations.

c. Western institutions carefully regulate the time when caring and treatment is provided to clients. Aboriginal people are much less concerned with the clock. Often, traditional Aboriginal healers provide healing ceremonies in the evenings when spiritual forces are believed to move about unobserved.

d. Among the Cree people, Euro-Aboriginal relationships have been established by various treaties. One expectation is that "white man's medicine" will always be provided, per a traditional understanding of the treaties' "medicine chest clause."

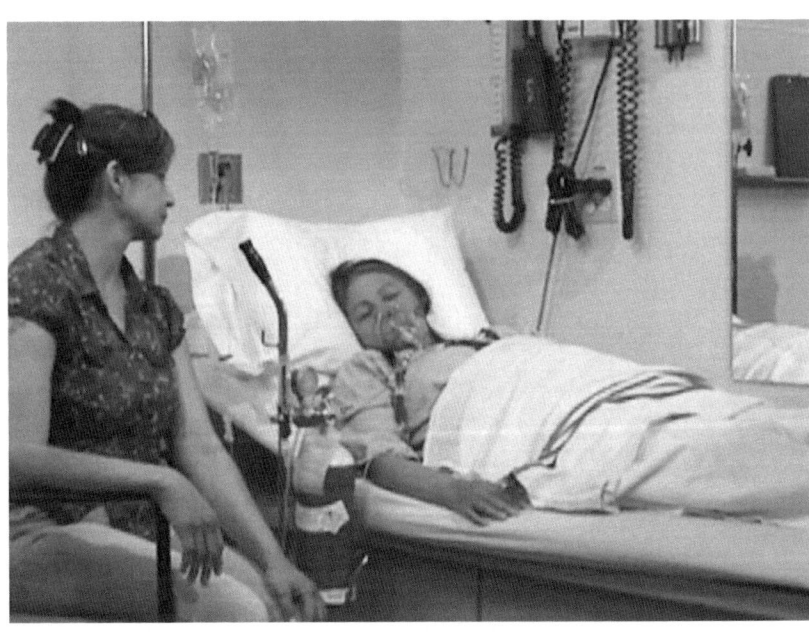

e. Cree people value independence of the person in their life-course and want medical intervention geared to that personal sense of what is right for the individual.

4. Decision Making for Health Care Issues and Caregiving

a. Among Aboriginal people, decision making is usually affected by the consensus of family members.

b. Caregiving is assigned first to the immediate family (daughter or son) or to the closest and most available relative, then to peers of the same or relatively similar age.

5. Aboriginal Beliefs, Values, and Health Care Outcome Expectations

a. Non-compliance/compliance is often dependent upon expectations. Western medicine is understood to act immediately or quickly. If this does not happen, the treatment is rejected and other traditional methods are often used.

b. It is known that traditional medicine through ceremony takes time to be effective.

c. Social and cultural roles may interfere with Western protocols, leading either to their rejection or non-compliance. Generally, adherence to tradition is considered more important than personal gain.

6. Unique Aboriginal End-of-Life Issues

a. Providing prognosis is not under the authority of physicians or health care professionals. End-of-life issues are controlled by the realm of the Spirit World through the spiritual leader or advisor. Non-direct communication is especially valued and respected among the Woodland Cree people in Wabasca. Generally, Aboriginal people prefer to maintain hope during interactions with those who are seriously ill.

b. Both Woodland and Plains Cree would prefer to be completely physically whole or complete at end-of-life to "walk on the path of their ancestors." For example, the right arm is considered to be especially important for power in a male, and legs need to be intact to walk this path. One should be very cautious about altering the body of the dying.

c. Death should not be divisive. It should, if at all possible, occur at home with caring people present. It should be "natural."

Module 2: Cultural Issues in Obtaining Consent (LEARN Model)

Listen *respectfully to the client's perception of the problem. Get the cultural story.*

Listen to the client's and family's views on end-of-life issues. Make special provisions when medical opinion must be filtered through translation. Determine how traditional the client's views are, and acknowledge that a biomedical approach may not always be appropriate.

Explain *your understanding of this family's cultural perspectives.*

Explain that consent forms for medical treatment give permission to professionals to undertake treatment. Clarify that the client and health provider should have come to an understanding of the implications of the consent form. Acknowledge that the translation of the consent was filtered and not fully conveyed.

Acknowledge *the impact of community on personal health compliance.*

Acknowledge that there are cultural implications of treatment to clients. Care should be taken that clients understand those implications.

Recommend *a culturally sensitive health care solution.*

Recommend that before surgery, both physician and family agree to a round-table discussion of the implications of treatment and consent. Discuss the cultural implications of treatment. Try to get a third party (designated hospital translator, client's peer, or Aboriginal healer), rather than a family member, to do the translation.

Negotiate *common ground that builds a competency bridge.*

Negotiate with the client and family as equals, with the intent to address as many of the treatment and cultural concerns as possible. Accept that cultural views may differ from biomedical views.

Module 2: Helpful Hints for Culturally Sensitive Care Plan Solutions that Consider Cultural Issues in Obtaining Consent

1. To what degree is the conflict in this film related to inadequate translation and/or to lack of cultural understanding?

Discussion points:

- Relatives of Cree people, especially those who are younger, are reluctant to give bad news. They may not believe that the doctor has the authority to make such prognoses. It may be that this played a role in the lack of discussion about possible leg removal.

- Had the doctor known the importance of walking whole in the realm of one's ancestors, he might have taken a different approach.

2. How was the consent form communicated, and how did the patient and family understand it?

Discussion points:

- A key issue is what the patient understood at the time of the intervention. If she was not aware of the difficulties that might arise, it is not acceptable that the physician utilize a consent form's fine print to carry out the operation. Communication seems to have been lacking in this case.

- Information had to be conveyed in the ER, and it had to be understood by the relative of the patient. It is not clear if the relative of the patient did not understand, if she changed her mind, or if the translation was poor.

3. What is the conflict in the film between what might be called artificial (biomedical) and natural views of life?

Discussion points:

- According to a traditional or natural view of the world, the removal of a limb seriously compromises a person moving on in the same status and with the same vigour on the pathways of the forbears as was enjoyed in this life. The complete body is necessary for wholeness.

4. What is the conflict between traditional Aboriginal views of afterlife and those derived from Christian culture?

Discussion points:

- Cree perceptions are that the next world is much like this one, without the problems associated with one's life here.

- Christians believe that the soul lives on, but the person's relationship with his or her physical body in the afterlife is less clear.

5. **Why is it not appropriate in Aboriginal culture to speak of someone's demise, even if medically it might be imminent?**

Discussion points:

- Only those who have been gifted to discern the other world (medicine people and spiritual people) can speak with any authority about "it."

- Health care professionals are not regarded as having these abilities and hence should not speak about anyone's death.

6. **Discuss the Aboriginal perspective of the future. How does this perspective compare to the Western perspective? What does this comparison reveal about Aboriginal views about one's use of words?**

Discussion points:

- In comparison with the Western perspective, Aboriginal viewpoints are generally far less concerned about the future. They regard the past and the present as the most important elements of time.

- Western science and culture is based on a thorough integration of past, present, and future.

- Aboriginal thinkers sometimes reject the confidence with which some speak of knowing the future.

7. **Aboriginal peoples place a great emphasis on listening. How can health professionals facilitate this?**

Discussion points:

- Many observers have noted the Aboriginal reluctance to speak on complicated topics. This is because most people have been taught that they should not speak unless they are an authority on a topic. On health matters, it is often the case that an Aboriginal person will emphasize listening to all relevant information before making a decision. This makes it appear that "silence is consent," when it is not.

- The health care system can facilitate the cultural importance of listening by setting up talking circles or sessions with a number of relatives present at which they can be urged to express their concerns. This will make the decision-making process much more comfortable for Aboriginal peoples.

Module 2: Cultural Understanding (BRIDGES Tool)

Insight into the values, beliefs, and attitudes of clients brings a deeper awareness of cultural perspectives. BRIDGES helps us gain deeper cultural understanding.

Beliefs, Values, Norms: Crisis situations in health call for the return to old values and the reaffirmation of Aboriginal beliefs. Very often these beliefs, values, and norms are clothed in Christian terms and concerns. However, such situations call for family and band loyalties, too.

Roles and Relationships with Family/Relatives: Group consciousness plays an important role among Aboriginal peoples of all ancestral lines. Generally, the closer one is to being a peer of the person, the more authority one will have to comprehend what should be done.

Identify Language, Literacy, Communication: Each family and community is apt to have selective attitudes toward health care. The language and communication means that individuals use indicates the level of importance placed on traditional views. It helps to listen closely in those situations, for there are often precise words associated with the person's future embedded in discussions.

Decision Making Methods/Practices: Family members who are closest to the ill person have a unique and powerful place in care, and they often "run interference" between the ill and the professional establishment. Decisions are made on the basis of the person's values, not on the basis of what the institution requires. In this case, the surgeon insisted on his prerogative to operate based on an earlier and perhaps vague approval. It is critical that decision making take the client's position into consideration.

Group, Community, Organizations: In this community, elderly women play a key role, and they are regarded as teachers of the next generation. It is important that their role is maintained so that younger members of the community continue to acknowledge their position in the community, even if they are ill. The Elder's status also affects the roles that younger members play when mediating between Elders and health care professionals.

Extraordinary Issues in Health (end-of-life, childbirth, etc.): The health care system's effect of adjusting social status (the assumption is that all individuals are equal) can inflict stress both on the caregiver and the community. Sensitivity to this issue will aid greatly in professional care.

Share Understanding of Cultures, Reach Common Ground, and Compromise: It is important to be aware of these norms, beliefs, and values and to develop a kind of common ground with the client regarding how the counselling professional creates a treatment plan. Engaging in discussion with the person's peers in the community or with the family will go a long way toward eliminating conflict about a therapeutic treatment plan.

Module 3: Cultural Issues in Compliance (LEARN Model)

Listen *respectfully to the client's perception of the problem. Get the cultural story.*

Listen to the client's and family's views on end-of-life issues. Make special provisions when medical opinion must be filtered through translation. Determine how traditional the client's views are, and acknowledge that a biomedical approach may not always be appropriate.

Explain *your understanding of this family's cultural perspectives.*

Explain that consent forms for medical treatment give permission to the physician to undertake treatment. Clarify that the client and health provider should have come to an understanding of the implications of the consent form. Acknowledge that the translation of the consent was filtered and not fully conveyed.

Acknowledge *the impact of community on personal health compliance.*

Acknowledge that there are cultural implications of treatment to clients. Care should be taken that clients understand those implications. Be aware that translation may be filtered by the translator.

Recommend *a culturally sensitive health care solution.*

Recommend that before a care plan has been accepted, both the medical and counselling team and the family agree to a round-table discussion of the implications of treatment and consent. Discuss the cultural implications of treatment. If translation is necessary, try to get a third party (designated hospital translator, client's peer, or Aboriginal healer) to do the translation.

Negotiate *common ground that builds a competency bridge.*

Negotiate with the client and family as equals, with the intent to address as many of the treatment and cultural concerns as possible. Accept that cultural views may differ from biomedical views.

Module 3: Helpful Hints for Culturally Sensitive Care Plan Solutions that Consider Cultural Issues in Compliance

1. How are traditional healers (known as gifted people) regarded in Aboriginal communities? How does this impact the healers' health?

Discussion points:

- Traditional healers (ceremonialists) are regarded very highly in Aboriginal communities because their skills are believed to have been bestowed on them from beyond for the benefit of the community. They are "gifted," which means they have some skill or benefit needed by the community.

- Some ceremonies are regarded as "medicinal," that is, they provide health and therapeutic value to the participants.

2. What intergenerational differences can be seen in the film? In what way is it possible that the importance of traditional views may not be known or understood by another generation?

Discussion points:

- The granddaughter is concerned only with her grandfather's continuing physical existence. A ceremonialist lives not to exist, however, but to serve his community. That takes priority in his mind, even above his own survival.

- The generational difference is demonstrated by the importance given to traditional ways. Many young Aboriginal people, raised in an urban environment, have not experienced the sophisticated ceremonial life on the reserve and thus cannot immediately identify with it.

- The grandfather appears to be much less concerned with the "future" than the granddaughter since she has been raised to think of the future as a real element of life. Her grandfather does not consider the notion of the "future" to be at all important in the matter. They may not understand each other's views.

3. To what degree do Cree people respect the individuals' rights to define their own lives?

Discussion points:

- The Cree community traditionally held that the individual was a necessary and complete part of "the people." Individual choices about how they would relate to the group seldom differed from the norms of the community. Thus, traditional Cree notions were that the person should be allowed as much freedom within the community as their position and status allowed. The community would not interfere in an individual's life unless she or he were in danger. The assumption is that no one from the community will step beyond community values.

- The granddaughter's logic is that grandfather should look after himself first, in effect stepping outside his position within the community. It is highly unlikely that a traditional Elder would do that.

4. How does Cree culture assert the integrity of the Elders' personal life? At what point should a family member step in to assist with support?

Discussion points:

- Matters of health are regarded as private and personal, with others intervening only if requested or when it is evident that the Elder is in trouble. As long as the grandfather believes he is doing what is right for his community, no one will step in to help. It is a different matter if and when he asks for help.
- Someone who is the grandfather's peer (i.e., his sister or brother or older relative (uncle) or a fellow ceremonialist) should assist with support.

5. What is the balance between body, mind, and spirit in Aboriginal culture?

Discussion points:

- The Cree understanding of such issues is quite different from that of Westerners. Western philosophy separates the person into mind and body, with the soul being a Christian theological addition. Cree notions accept four equal elements in a person's being: spirit, body, emotions, and mind—all of them necessarily in balance for a "whole" person.
- Many Cree people live in both systems of understanding, but one has to be aware of the traditional view because elderly people often affirm it in their attitudes. Moreover, as people age, they sometimes return to traditional views.

6. Do Aboriginal people make a distinction between a "traditional" disease and "white man's" disease? What impact does this have on diagnosis and treatment?

Discussion points:

- Yes, traditionalists will often speak about "white man's" disease and "Cree" disease, defining the first as diseases identified by Western science and the latter as problems that have been around for millennia among the people.
- They may not always be convinced of the validity of Western diseases, or they may hold that they came with the first European immigrants and have been very difficult for Aboriginal peoples to cope with.
- Diagnosis and compliance is sometimes compromised by those who do not place much confidence in Western medicine.

7. Is there any indication that the Elder's illness is the result of "bad medicine," that is, medicine set against the Elder by someone unhappy with his influence?

Discussion points:

- Traditional communities accepted that someone with spiritual power could send "bad medicine" against another member of the community, or outside it, over some emotionally charged issue. It is, however, usual for this kind of medicine to come quickly, not as the result of a long-term illness or chronic condition.

- Traditionally, "bad medicine" does not include "Western" types of diseases.

Module 3: Cultural Understanding (BRIDGES Tool)

Insight into the values, beliefs, and attitudes of clients brings a deeper awareness of cultural perspectives. BRIDGES helps us gain deeper understanding.

Beliefs, **Values, Norms**: Some roles/positions in the community trump all other concerns. The elderly, in particular, are sensitive to their role in the community as character builders and spiritual advisors. Theirs is a position that few others would attempt to take on themselves, and it plays a key role in personal notions of value and importance.

Roles and Relationships with Family/Relatives: Very often many cultures emphasize the place of family and group in all areas of life. Health care is critical in Cree culture because of the value placed on the aged.

Identify Language, Literacy, Communication: Even delivery style can indicate how acculturated an individual is to Western ways, as the young woman demonstrates. Traditional folk "read" how a person talks and draw conclusions about how sensitive professionals are to Aboriginal ways of thinking.

Decision Making Methods/Practices: Cultural issues divide many peoples, and the health care system must grapple with the fact that critical decisions about compliance have to be subject to the person's role in the community. Discussions about compliance and cultural roles did not happen in this scenario.

Group, Community, Organizations: Many elderly people value wisdom and community standing much higher than wealth or social position. Community perceptions are more important to the ceremonialist than his own health.

Extraordinary Issues in Health (end-of-life, childbirth, etc.): One's place in the community is understood to be one's gift to the community, so that role comes with great responsibility. Elders have a "modelling" role to play for young people.

Share Understanding of Cultures, Reach Common Ground, and Compromise: Sensitivity to cultural values at critical times like this will enable counselling professionals to provide more effective care. Reaching common ground is not easy, but it will provide a much more wholesome situation for everyone.

RESOURCE MATERIALS

Alberta Online Encyclopedia. The making of Treaty 8 in Canada's Northwest. Retrieved July 13, 2009, from http://www.albertasource.ca/treaty8/eng/default.htm

Hampton, M., Baydala, A., Bourassa, C., McKay-McNabb, K., Placsko, C., Goodwill, K., et al. (2010). Completing the circle: Elders speak about end-of-life care with Aboriginal families in Canada. *Journal of Palliative Care, 26*(1), 6–14.

Hendrie, H. C., Hall, K. S., Pillay, N., Rodgers, D., Prince, C., Norton, J., et al. (1993). Alzheimer's disease is rare in Cree. *International Psychogeriatrics, 5*(1), 5–14. http://dx.doi.org/10.1017/S1041610293001358

Indian and Northern Affairs Canada. Indian residential schools. Retrieved July 13, 2009, from http://www.aadnc-aandc.gc.ca/ai/rqpi/index-eng.asp

Jilek, W. G. (1992). *Indian healing: Shamanic ceremonialism in the Pacific Northwest today.* Surrey, BC: Hancock House Publishers, Ltd.

Kelly, L., & Minty, A. (2007). End-of-life issues for Aboriginal clients. A literature review. *Canadian Family Physician Medecin de Famille Canadien, 53*(9), 1459–1465.

Young, D., Ingram, G., & Swartz, L. (1989). *Cry of the eagle: Encounters with a Cree healer.* Toronto: University of Toronto Press.

Appendix C

Francophone Cultural Perspectives

1. Francophone Protocols of Interaction

    a. French-speaking communities across the country, including Alberta, Saskatchewan, and Manitoba and farther east into Ontario and Quebec, have emotional lines that link them to a special part of who they are. For some, the connection is directly with Quebec, where the resources and the inspiration for francophone culture is the catalyst for the rest of the country. At the same time, the Roman Catholic Church is a long-embraced cultural institution even if some religious ardour has abated. So, counselling professionals should pay special attention to family and religious connections.

    b. In traditional culture, the father was the head and the public face of the family. All issues of significance to the family required his approval. This condition has greatly diminished over time; nevertheless, elderly members of the community continue to preserve francophone culture even today. This suggests that health care professionals need to ascertain who is the most respected and honoured member of the family, since that individual will retain considerable responsibility in health care decisions. Families may accept that these responsibilities are delegated because of distance or other factors, but knowing the nuances of family hierarchy will ease matters in a crisis situation.

    c. Family consultations will usually designate who will speak for the ill person: usually the person who lives closest or who is nearest in kinship relationship.

2. Francophone Language and Communication

    a. Given that immigration has brought different dialects of French to Canada, there may be some problems of intergenerational communications. Younger people may have problems understanding those whose French derives from a different cultural milieu.

    b. Our study found considerable difference in attitude toward resuscitation protocols between older francophones (seventy-plus years) and their now senior children. The older people were opposed to resuscitation simply because they were confident that their religious beliefs sustained them. Their children were not so confident and were reluctant to "let them go."

    c. Language reversion sometimes occurs to those who have a serious illness, such as a stroke or brain injury. Health care professionals who work with francophone populations may likely encounter the phenomenon and should be aware of the inherent complications for health care provision that it entails.

3. Provision of Health Care by Community and Organizations

   a. Francophone organizations show great sensitivity to lack of facilities in French. Especially in a service sector like health, where a high value is placed on communication, community response to lack of proper linguistic services can generate considerable controversy. In environments where the francophone population makes up a significant minority, health administration will need to address any lack of French-speaking health care workers.

   b. Francophone populations may be much better organized and utilize the system in a much more sophisticated manner than do many other ethnic groups. In many cases, the older members of society have worked hard to ensure that French language services are available in critical areas. Given Canada's official bilingualism, the claim for French services may put strains on the often-unilingual state of many agencies. Health care professionals who work in francophone-dominant regions will do well to acquire the French language.

4. Francophone Beliefs, Values, and Health Care Outcome Expectations

   a. Our research revealed that older seniors found solace in their religion (Roman Catholicism was the dominant religion in the region we studied). Priests and lay workers can be called upon to assist families at this difficult time, and elderly clients appreciate that support. Facilitating that support will add to the health provider's status in the community.

   b. Identifying the client's religious affiliation will help with providing spiritual care.

5. Unique End-of-Life Issues in the Francophone Community

   a. Although personal directives have not been embraced by the community, there appears to be growing interest in the procedure among the oldest members of the community. The personal directive is regarded as a way of reducing extended life-courses when quality of life may scarcely be present.

   b. There is some resistance among younger people to advance the cause of personal directives because they value the elders in the community.

Module 4: Language Diversity in Health Care (LEARN Model)

Listen *respectfully to the client's perception of the problem. Get the cultural story.*

Listen as the daughter contends that someone should have been available to communicate with her mother in French.

Explain *your understanding of this family's cultural perspectives.*

Explain to the daughter the difficulty in providing completely bilingual health care personnel at all times, and add that whenever possible translation services will be sought. Explain to health care providers that language reversion may occur in clients with dementia. Explain to the young nurse that she should have checked the client's chart before attempting to turn her.

Acknowledge *the importance of language diversity in client care and service.*

Acknowledge the importance of communication in providing health care service.

Recommend *a culturally sensitive health care solution.*

Recommend that language reversion should be documented in the chart and that, whenever possible, bilingual personnel or translators should be available to elderly francophone clients, especially during health crises. Recommend that the young nurse should have checked the chart before providing care.

Negotiate *common ground that builds a competency bridge.*

Negotiate with the daughter who attends the client to determine what issues there may be so that health providers can deal as professionally as possible with the situation. Indicate that translation services will be accessed whenever possible.

Module 4: Helpful Hints for Culturally Sensitive Care Plan Solutions that Consider Language Diversity in Health Care

1. What are the indicators of language reversion?

Discussion points:

- Language reversion can arise after a brain trauma, such as that brought on by mini strokes or dementia. The language portion of the brain returns to the earliest language development, one associated with early childhood. Other areas of memory may also be affected.

2. How can psychologists respond to such a situation effectively?

Discussion points:

- Even if the health care professional is not aware of language reversion, the client's inability to converse in his or her second language will become apparent. Signs include lack of response to simple queries and unanswered references to relatives and friends. The medical history may not contain information about the first language, so family will need to provide some assistance.
- Translators may be engaged.
- It might be helpful to determine ahead of time the language the elderly person spoke early in childhood and document that information to the medical record.

3. How did hospital procedures contribute to the crisis in this situation?

Discussion points:

- Emergency situations in care and change of shifts came together to make this case problematic.
- Communication between staff was compromised.

4. How would cultural training have helped in the situation?

Discussion points:

- Cultural training could have made all staff aware of the possibility of language reversion.

5. Is there any evidence that anyone had documented language reversion on the chart?

Discussion points:

- No. The issue apparently had never been discussed regarding this case.

Module 4: Cultural Understanding (BRIDGES Tool)

Insight into the values, beliefs, and attitudes of clients brings a deeper awareness of their cultural perspectives. BRIDGES helps us gain deeper cultural understanding.

Beliefs, Values, Norms: Many communities place more stress on some beliefs than other communities do. Strongly held beliefs are a source of richness and cultural diversity, but they can also lead to major implications when dealing with some critical issues that rely on communications, like health. Then beliefs can challenge major systems.

Roles and Relationships with Family/Relatives: The role of the French language is critical in this family, and it provides a solid cultural base upon which decision making will be made. Communication is a fundamental feature of francophone cultural life and plays a key role in crisis situations.

Identify Language, Literacy, Communication: Language diversity has always been a sensitive issue in Canada, and this case reflects how cultures diverge on its importance. The francophone community treasures the role of French in family life, and physician sensitivity about language will provide better care.

Decision Making Methods/Practices: Hospital protocols may make sense within the management system of the institution, but they are often unresponsive to the nuances of care. Even emergency decisions may be a problem. The cultural side of care has to be considered if care is to be properly carried out.

Group, Community, Organizations: In this situation, for this family, adequacy of the system was found wanting because it did not take language reversion into consideration.

Extraordinary Issues in Health (end-of-life, childbirth, etc.): Language reversion is a common phenomenon among the elderly who have had strokes. Awareness of the potential problems that result from language reversion will pay off with better health care.

Share Understanding of Cultures, Reach Common Ground, and Compromise: Sensitivity about language is a foundational value in Canada, especially among some communities. Making the attempt to mediate problems related to language and communication within institutions will help people who speak different languages to work together.

Module 7: Challenging Cultural Norms (LEARN Model)

Listen *respectfully to the client's perception of the problem. Get the cultural story.*

Listen to the mother's wishes for end-of-life care. She is a woman of considerable religious faith and wishes her death to be in keeping with her desire to pass peacefully into the afterlife. She wants heroic, end-of-life interventions to be minimized. By documenting her wishes in a personal directive, she hopes to reduce stress and anxiety in the family.

Explain *your understanding of this family's religious perspectives.*

Explain that valid personal directives will be followed by hospital personnel for end-of-life care. If a personal directive is not in place, hospital protocol will be followed.

Acknowledge *the impact of religious perspectives on end-of-life care.*

Acknowledge that hospital protocols at end-of-life may not coincide with what the client may have wanted.

Recommend *a culturally sensitive health care solution.*

Recommend that family members be aware of any personal directives and end-of-life wishes and communicate these to health care providers as soon as possible.

Negotiate *common ground that builds a competency bridge.*

Negotiate that end-of-life care will be provided in accordance with a written personal directive.

Module 7: Helpful Hints for Culturally Sensitive Care Plan Solutions that Consider Challenging Cultural Norms

1. **How much does the woman's concern about end-of-life relate to her experience with hospitals?**

Discussion points:

- The death of her brother clearly has made the problem of end-of-life protocols critical to her. She experienced firsthand the traumas associated with intubation and general hospital protocols for a severely ill client.

2. **Why is it important to the mother to have a personal directive as it relates to her children and family members?**

Discussion points:

- For her, the important issue is dying with dignity and without prolonged emergency procedures. The personal directive is seen as a way to keep her children from entering conflicts among themselves over her death. Her religious beliefs are defined by the notion that God will call her home and there is no need to delay her death unnecessarily.

3. **How are francophone ethnicity, language, and religion intertwined? To what degree can this be generalized to all francophones?**

Discussion points:

- In our study, Franco-Albertans appeared to be very much concerned for the continuing influence of French language and culture in the province. There was a strong conviction that everything had to be done to retain the elderly as effective representatives of a lively French culture. This contributed to a reluctance on the part of older sons and daughters of these pioneer people to let them go. They were reluctant to have them write personal directives. On the other hand, among the most elderly, there was a strong connection between religion, culture, and end-of-life commitments. Their attitudes were more clearly defined by their religious views.

- It is unlikely that all francophone speakers are dedicated members of a church and have such convictions about end-of-life. The Christian church is now so diversified that only traditional and conservative Christians might fit this situation.

4. **Do hospital procedures override religious views when a client does not have a personal directive?**

Discussion points:

- Yes. Hospitals are required by law to undertake every life-saving protocol available, including emergency procedures in this case.

- Religious views cannot trump these protocols unless there is a legal document specifying otherwise. However, religious views might enter into the discussion in the absence of an authorizing document for surgery. Sometimes relatives are not familiar with the implications of signing an emergency acceptance document.

Module 7: Cultural Understanding (BRIDGES Tool)

Insight into the values, beliefs, and attitudes of clients brings a deeper awareness of cultural perspectives. BRIDGES helps us gain a deeper cultural understanding.

Beliefs, Values, Norms: The move to hospital for many deaths has changed the dynamics of beliefs; even the professional goal to "do no harm" may conflict with cultural values adopted by some communities. In this case, the stress arising from conflict can be mediated by an awareness of the problem.

Roles and Relationships with Family/Relatives: In this culture, the sibling relationship assisted the sister to know what her brother wanted, an implication of close community/family values.

Identify Language, Literacy, Communication: The emphasis here was less on Christian beliefs clashing with the hospital system and more on the desire to maintain family dominance over end-of-life issues. That the family wishes to control what happens at end-of-life, in this case, tells us that identity resides within a complex of values undergirded by Catholic faith and community solidarity.

Decision Making Methods/Practices: Separation from family and community at end-of-life was a key value in this case, and it also holds for many within the larger society. Even the move from a rural community to an urban centre for treatment poses problems. Health care professionals need to be aware of this dimension of rural community life and factor it into decision making.

Group, Community, Organizations: In this family, support may be provided by religious leaders and the community.

Extraordinary Issues in Health (end-of-life, childbirth, etc.): Strong religious belief sometimes trumps health protocols. Not all people in North America are willing to accept the process of acculturation implied in our health care system, with its dominance of English and its insistence on preserving life at all costs.

Share Understanding of Cultures, Reach Common Ground, and Compromise: It is important to be aware that these norms, beliefs, and values develop in different ways with different outcomes for many minority groups. A common ground can be reached by showing some awareness of the issue in discussions with principal members of the family.

RESOURCE MATERIALS

Association Canadienne de Soins Palliatifs & La Fondation GlaxoSmithKline. *Guide des aidants.* Retrieved June 12, 2009, from http://acsp.net//adiants-naturels.aspx

Deachman, M., & Howell, D. (1994). *Soins de soutien à domicile: Guide à l'intention de clients gravement malades et de leur famille.* Montreal: Édition BASF Knoll-Pharma Inc.

Deachman, M., & Howell, D. (2002). *Supportive care at home: A guide for seriously ill clients and their families.* Saint-Laurent, QC: Abbott Laboratories Ltd. http:// libraries.phsa.ca/list?mlt=Diabetes+handouts+for+patients+and+families&q=&p=1&date_facet=2000s

del Ser, T., Barba, R., Morin, M. M., Domingo, J., Cemillan, C., Pondal, M., & Vivancos, J. (2005). Evolution of cognitive impairment after stroke and risk factors for delayed progression. *Stroke, 36*(12), 2670–2675. http://dx.doi.org/10.1161/01.STR.0000189626.71033.35

Fainsinger, R., & Young, C. (1991). Cognitive failure in a terminally ill client. *Journal of Pain and Symptom Management, 6*(8), 492–494. http://dx.doi.org/10.1016/0885-3924(91)90007-Q

Roth, E. J., Fink, K., Cherney, L. R., & Hall, K. D. (1997). Reversion to a previously learned foreign accent after stroke. *Archives of Physical Medicine and Rehabilitation, 78*(5), 550–552. http://dx.doi.org/10.1016/S0003-9993(97)90176-3

Appendix D

Chinese Cultural Perspectives

1. Traditional Chinese Protocols of Interaction

a. Public perceptions remain an important value for most Chinese families, and many will not display strong emotions outside the home or where they may be observed by others. Similarly, Chinese family values defer public discourse to male heads of family, with considerable effort expended to receive the older male's opinions on major decisions. Female spouses may be reluctant to provide illness details to health care professionals in deference to the oldest son, or a more educated daughter. There may be great latitude around this issue, depending on the length of time and experience of the family in Canada.

b. There remains a strong honouring of one's ancestral line, especially among Cantonese-speaking Chinese. Within the medical setting, this can be expressed as doing everything possible for one's elders. There is considerable reluctance in appearing to the community to be doing less than is possible for elder family members. In addition, many remain loyal to Buddhist traditions, even if they are not actively practiced.

c. A life-limiting prognosis may require a protocol that allows the individual to be as conscious as possible, since it is believed that transitions to the next life are best made in a state of conscious awareness.

d. Family members will ultimately look for the most authoritative person to be present at consultations. Among Mandarin speakers, this is the most senior available person. Among Cantonese speakers, the authority is the oldest and most respected male in the family.

e. Communal values play an essential role in personal life decisions.

2. Chinese Language and Communication

a. Even among Chinese people who immigrated many years ago, there may be significant problems in understanding English. Medical terms should be avoided as much as possible. Deference to a "white coat" may restrict attempts to clarify information.

b. The use of jokes to "break the ice" should be avoided until a long-standing relationship has formed. There is some cultural resistance to professionals who joke around.

c. Caution should be used in choosing who acts as translator, since there may be issues revealed that not all members of the family would like to have aired publicly. If at all possible, translators from outside the family should be avoided. It cannot be assumed that children of a second generation are able to speak the language effectively enough for a sophisticated exchange. Translation issues should be privately discussed with the leading family member at the outset of counselling.

    d. Elderly clients, especially when they are ill, prefer their original language to be spoken. If deterioration has taken place following a stroke, clients may revert to an original language, even if they have been perfectly bilingual all their lives.

3. Provision of Health Care by Community and Organizations

    a. Chinese cultural communities usually have communicators who know the community and its values well. They can be accepted as part of a team if the family is scattered or the lines of communication are not clear. In most cases, these individuals are respected for their position within the community and can be relied upon for information about family matters.

    b. Mandarin-speaking families may be less connected to community organizations than Cantonese speakers, as they may have emigrated from mainland China later and have integrated into the community less thoroughly. They may also have fewer family members in Canada, or the family members may be spread out across the country. For these people, the allegiance to family may be less defined than it is for Cantonese speakers. In many cases, a spokesperson will emerge during consultations.

    c. Western institutions are carefully regulated with regard to time and type of nutrition. Chinese people may be less concerned about such rules. Indeed, they may arrange for "proper" food to be brought in for hospitalized clients. They may also be less concerned with protocols of bathing because of beliefs regarding the proper times for hot and cold applications. Some flexibility on these matters may help to reduce tensions.

    d. Chinese people are usually very much committed to the promise of "free" health care in Canada and resist suggestions of curbing treatment because of cost. Indeed, the suggestion to stop treatment may be regarded as discriminatory by them. It is better that discussions remain related to matters of client comfort and convey a caring response to a situation.

4. Decision Making for Health Care Issues and Caregiving

    a. Ultimate decision making rests with the eldest son, or the oldest and most respected member of the family. This holds for Cantonese speakers in particular, but this tradition is also found among older Mandarin speakers.

    b. Caregiving is assigned first to an immediate family member (daughter or son) or to the closest, most available relative, and then to peers of the same/similar age.

    c. Serious illness will bring the extended family into discussions. In the absence of family, a community member of some standing may be called upon to assist.

5. Chinese Beliefs, Values, and Health Care Outcome Expectations

    a. Non-compliance/compliance may be dependent upon the perceived status of the health care professional—that is, the higher the medical credentials, the more authority is attributed to him or her by the client. There may also be a perception that male health care personnel have more authority than females.

b. Discussions with family may reveal that alternative systems of medicine are also being used. Self-selection of therapies has a long tradition in China, and this practice continues in Canada.

c. Compliance ordinarily will be the case due to the Chinese value of the family member, or the ancestral commitment, or respect for the medical authority.

6. Unique Chinese End-of-Life Issues

a. Effective and elaborate rituals at end-of-life have considerable history in Chinese cultures, and there is a great emphasis placed on proper protocols for this time of life. Traditionally, the status and position of the individual determined how death would be observed. Death calls for a community response, and the assumption is that everything possible has been done to maintain the person in a viable living state until departure. There is some reluctance to create a personal directive because that suggests that the family will not "do the right thing" as death draws near. No family wants to be remembered by the community for not "doing the right thing."

b. The concern for an honourable transition into the world of the ancestors causes some friction with hospital protocols related to personal directives. To ask a family to commit to "no code" is to require them to submit the honouring of their esteemed loved one to the mechanical protocols of a modern institution (i.e., to a system quite divorced from their ancestral sensitivities).

c. Even Chinese community members who are Christian may express traditional ancestral views concerning older members of the community. Death is an occasion for community cohesion; traditionally, rites were designed to send the deceased to the ancestral world with great ritual and ceremony.

Module 6: Generational Views on Personal Directives (LEARN Model)

Listen *respectfully to the client's perception of the problem. Get the cultural story.*

Listen to the Chinese mother as she is concerned with the medical circumstances surrounding the death of her brother in hospital. She disapproves of all the heroic medical interventions that were done to no avail. When it comes her time to die, she wants to go peacefully. She wants her eldest son to honour her by respecting her end-of-life wishes, which she intends to document in a personal directive.

Explain *your understanding of this family's perspective of personal directives.*

Explain that personal directives (living wills) state one's wishes for health care and medical treatment in the event that one is not able to make medical decisions by oneself sometime in the future. In the absence of a personal directive, those decisions must be made by the family or an appointed guardian. Personal directives are not traditional in Chinese culture.

Acknowledge *the generational gap in fulfilling end-of-life issues.*

Acknowledge the traditional role of eldest son as decision maker in such situations, and carry out only the procedures that are necessary until the son has been contacted. If contact with the eldest son cannot be made in time, then the next male relative is normally called. Be aware that the mother is going against the cultural tradition of the son having total decision-making responsibility should she be incapacitated.

Recommend *a culturally sensitive health care solution.*

Recommend that the son be fully aware of his mother's condition so he can authorize the treatment compatible with her wishes. Do not recommend treatment not consistent with her expressed wishes.

Negotiate *common ground that builds a competency bridge.*

Negotiate with the son regarding how he will abide by the personal directive set by his mother. He will be honouring her by respecting her wishes.

Module 6: Helpful Hints for Culturally Sensitive Solutions that Consider Generational Views on Personal Directives

1. **How typical is it for a Chinese mother to have a conversation about personal directives with her son? What does this say about her awareness of Canadian hospital procedures and the length of time she has been in Canada?**

   Discussion points:

   - Chinese women are usually reluctant to speak about issues relating to death, except with very close relatives. In this case she is speaking to her son, who will carry on the family honour. He is duty-bound to take his mother's wishes seriously. Still, the conversation is extraordinary, perhaps reflecting that the mother has been in Canada for some time and her son is used to her forthright speech.

   - She appears to be quite knowledgeable about hospital protocols in Canada.

2. **The mother makes her pleas on the basis of quality of life during the last moments of life. How can a counselling professional handle clients who are not as able to articulate their wishes for end-of-life treatment?**

   Discussion points:

   - Passing into the next world should not be fraught with difficulty for Chinese people. Many would like to experience an "auspicious" death, best reflected in a death that is not agonizing or difficult. Depending upon religious perspectives, a "difficult" death might portend unfortunate occurrences in the next existence. Most will not articulate this to health care professionals. It is best to suggest a plan for a calm and peaceful end, and to plan for that.

3. **What conflicts do you see between normal hospital procedures and the mother's desires?**

   Discussion points:

   - If she has no official document indicating a personal directive, the hospital will make every effort to maintain her on life support, despite the present plea to her son. If her son expressly asks that no extraordinary measures be taken, the hospital might continue the support until they are assured that nothing more can be done.

4. **What problems may arise with personal directives, even if they appear to represent the client's wishes?**

   Discussion points:

   - Hospitals may be reluctant to act on personal directives if there is any indication of contention in the family. A handwritten directive clearly cannot be used because the health care professional might believe it was written under duress. It is not likely that anything but a legally validated document would be acceptable. Even then, if there is strong disagreement among family members, it might not be acted upon.

5. **What is the conflict between traditional Chinese views of an afterlife and those deriving from Canadian culture?**

Discussion points:

- Chinese tradition may hold to some form of post-death existence, such as that held by Buddhist tradition, where the individual will be transformed into another being in the afterlife and be reborn into a new existence. Among some members of this community, the importance given to mental awareness indicates a preference for a state as conscious as possible—that is, not one in which painkillers act to cloud consciousness, ensuring that one is able to transmigrate easily to the next life, being fully conscious at all times.

- Canadian society is heavily influenced by Christian tradition, which sees this life as a stepping stone to a blissful paradise. The transition to that life does not require any awareness, so sedation is not limited by the desire to be conscious at the moments leading up to death.

6. **Had the discussion between the mother and son not taken place, what would have transpired?**

Discussion points:

- Had the mother not had this discussion, the son might necessarily agree to all emergency procedures and, indeed, would contend for them out of deference to community opinion.

Module 6: Cultural Understanding (BRIDGES Tool)

Insight into the values, beliefs, and attitudes of clients brings a deeper awareness of cultural perspectives. BRIDGES helps us gain deeper cultural understanding.

Beliefs, Values, Norms: All cultures have specific ways of dealing with death, and Chinese culture is no different. Generally there is great reluctance to raise issues relative to death because it will bring the experience closer. Obviously this will have implications for health care professionals as they try to deal with a dying loved one.

Roles and Relationships with Family/Relatives: In traditional Chinese culture, the role of speaking about end-of-life issues would not be assigned to a woman, even a senior woman. In North America, however, roles have evolved, partly because of the sparse nature of the community and the lack of male family members.

Identify Language, Literacy, Communication: In some cultures, words are believed to have power. Speaking of death, or discussing it, is not just bad form, it means the negativity of the experience somehow sticks to the person. The mother feels so strongly about her position that she speaks; she knows that the cultural health environment here will somehow bring things to pass that she does not want.

Decision Making Methods/Practices: Normally, Chinese males are entrusted with the role of leadership in all matters pertaining to the family. This is a cultural residue from Confucianism that stressed the cohesive nature of family life focused on the male line. This emphasis on family life and the male line is still maintained, but obviously living abroad has complicated its implementation.

Group, Community, Organizations: Solidarity within Chinese tradition is hard to establish because of the many influences on community life, but in this family, the mother wanted to make sure that nothing like what happened to her brother would happen to her.

Extraordinary Issues in Health (end-of-life, childbirth, etc.): Ideally, passing to the next life should be easy and without loss of awareness until the moment of departure. This way, one is welcomed to the next world while still in a conscious state. Adjusting personal endings to reflect this belief is a matter of great concern for people of Chinese descent living in the West.

Share Understanding of Cultures, Reach Common Ground, and Compromise: It is important to be aware of these norms, beliefs, and values and develop common ground with clients because situations can develop in which there is great antagonism with the health care system. Health care professionals need to be aware of the diversity of views about death within the community.

Final Evaluation: Cultural Issues in End-of-Life Care (LEARN Model)

Listen *respectfully to the client's perception of the problem. Get the cultural story.*

Listen to the children who want to be loyal to their father's ancestral tradition, which in this context means providing him with all medical procedures at the hospital's disposal. They wish to be "good children" and not be known to their fellow Chinese community members as children who did not properly respect their father's life. They feel they have no choice but not to agree to "no code." Also, listen to determine who speaks for the family line (oldest son, uncle, elder) in decision-making matters.

Explain *your understanding of this family's cultural perspective.*

As a health professional, explain to the children that you would prefer to speak about giving their father the most humane treatment as a measure of your respect for him. Indicate that as he is rapidly declining and not responding to treatment, alleviating pain and providing comfort is key at his stage.

Acknowledge *the influence of cultural perspectives on end-of-life care.*

Acknowledge the children's concern for maintaining ancestral respect and explain how that differs from the goals of an acute-care hospital.

Recommend *a culturally sensitive health care solution.*

Recommend that psychologists should focus on providing the best care under the circumstances. Prevent the conversation from dwelling on the palliative, no-code provision.

Negotiate *common ground that builds a competency bridge.*

Negotiate from a position of solidarity with the family, as if you are a proxy member of the family trying to handle a difficult situation. Maintaining family cohesion at this time is very important, especially in the light of ancestral honouring.

Final Evaluation: Helpful Hints for Culturally Sensitive Solutions that Consider Cultural Issues in End-of-Life Care

1. How does polarization develop between the family and the doctor?

Discussion points:

- The crucial issue of whether or not to prolong protocols in the case of the elderly father was the main point of contention between the family and the doctor. From the family's perspective, the no-code issue became the central factor in the approach of the hospital and the doctor to their father's care.

- The commitment to doing everything for one's relative is set over against the protocols of the hospital.

2. How might the doctor have minimized the confrontation earlier on?

Discussion points:

- The professional could have avoided this polarization by stressing the quality of care the hospital was providing to the client, along with an emphasis on maintaining him in a comfortable and pain-free condition.

- The transference to an extended-care facility could have been achieved without affecting the no-code provision.

3. What is at stake culturally for the family as they try to negotiate with the doctor? What is the decision-making hierarchy in this Chinese family?

Discussion points:

- Traditional Chinese values maintain the ancestral line; this is basic to each family member's own sense of proper existence.

- If the Chinese community perceives that the children have done less than provide their father with all life-prolonging treatments, they will be denounced by the faithful. To be respectful, the children must do everything in their power to honour his life. In the traditional family, honouring one's ancestors is honouring oneself and one's linkage to the family's great relatives.

- The eldest son is considered the authority for all decision making with regard to honour and preserving the respect of the ancestral line.

4. How could the medical condition have been explained in a simpler way?

Discussion points:

- The difficulty began when the doctor used medical talk instead of stressing the father's inability to eat, as well as his general deterioration. She could then have discussed how treatment in a long-term facility could emphasize dignity and calm for his last days.

5. What do you see happening in the institution regarding the doctor's response to the family?

Discussion points:

- The family might complain about the doctor's treatment, in which case she will likely be removed from the case. Her relationship with the family is probably beyond repair.

6. How might the Chinese community respond had the family said nothing to the doctor? Does the physician's attitude while working with the family reflect an appreciation of the elder client's community status?

Discussion points:

- If community members were aware of the circumstances, they might be critical of the son for not "sticking up" for ancestral values. On the other hand, they would have to know all the details of the case.

- What is at stake here is the son's duty to his ancestors.

- The doctor showed no familiarity with Chinese ancestral beliefs. Had she been aware, she might have stressed the importance of providing him the best and most humane care for the remainder of his life.

7. Are there any options for handling the no-code protocol in palliative care units that could have been brought up at this time?

Discussion points:

- Such institutions maintain no code because they focus on palliative care. The emphasis should be on humane care and respect for the life that is left. The doctor's theme might have shifted more properly toward better care than to the no-code issue.

8. Discuss the notion of "best care" from the perspective of the family and that of the physician.

Discussion points:

- The notion of "best care" allows for discussion about which elements of care the family considers most important. Care could perhaps shift to maintaining the client in a conscious state as long as possible, so that the family could spend quality time with the father before his demise. In that case, the family could also focus on honouring him after death, in a manner that conveys as much honour as possible.

- The doctor might have shifted the discussion to honouring the father in the last days of his life, which would link to the Confucian value of respect for the ancestral line.

Final Evaluation: Cultural Understanding (BRIDGES Tool)

Insight into the values, beliefs, and attitudes of clients brings a deeper awareness of cultural perspectives. BRIDGES helps us gain deeper cultural understanding.

Beliefs, Values, Norms: Conflicts between systems in health care can result in major confrontations, and many cultures are extremely sensitive regarding seniors' end-of-life. This is a case in which there is direct conflict between the protocols of the hospital and several important beliefs held by the young people.

Roles and Relationships with Family/Relatives: In this culture, the eldest male had to make the final decision, and clearly he found it very difficult to deal with the protocols communicated by the doctor.

Identify Language, Literacy, Communication: It is evident that information and emphases in communication are just as important as content. Here the conversation was hijacked by the issue of "no code." The case also demonstrates the difficulty in establishing procedures when clients cannot express their own views.

Decision Making Methods/Practices: In this culture, the decision making had implications for how the young people would be viewed in their community. Decisions cannot be made so that the living appear to slight the dead. Hence, no decision about hospital protocols will be tolerated if it results in a "less than best" death.

Group, Community, Organizations: In this family, support comes from the community at large, and also from elderly members of the family who cannot be present.

Extraordinary Issues in Health (end-of-life, childbirth, etc.): Traditionally, no overt planning would be done in the case of a prolonged, suffering death, for the simple reason that death is regarded negatively. To plan for it is to hurry it along. The result is the rejection of Western, advanced-planning options.

Share Understanding of Cultures, Reach Common Ground, and Compromise: It is important to be aware of these norms, beliefs, and values and develop common ground. The best option is to stress the positive experience for the loved one in certain types of hospitals and to leave the issue of "no code" aside. Here, common experiences can help, especially those of the health care professional who has encountered other related cases.

RESOURCE MATERIALS

Kramer, E. J., Kwong, K., Lee, E., & Chung, H. (2002). Cultural factors influencing the mental health of Asian Americans. *Western Journal of Medicine, 176*(4), 227–231.

Lai, D. W., & Surood, S. (2009). Chinese health beliefs of older Chinese in Canada. *Journal of Aging and Health, 21*(1), 38–62. http://dx.doi.org/10.1177/0898264308328636

Ngo-Metzger, Q., Legedza, A. T., & Phillips, R. S. (2004). Asian Americans' reports of their health care experiences: Results of a national survey. *Journal of General Internal Medicine, 19*(2), 111–119. http://dx.doi.org/10.1111/j.1525 -1497.2004.30143.x

Ruan, S. (2008). About a boy: A piece of my mind. *Journal of the American Medical Association, 300*(7), 771–772. http:// dx.doi.org/10.1001/jama.300.7.771

Tom, L. A. S. H. (2001). Health and health care for Chinese-American elders. In G. Yeo (ed.), *Curriculum in ethnogeriatrics: Chinese* (2nd ed). *Core curriculum and ethnic specific modules. Health and health care for Chinese-American elders.* Retrieved October 30, 2014, from http://web.stanford.edu/group/ethnoger/chinese.html

Yue, K. K. (2005). People of Chinese descent. In N. Waxler-Morrison, J. M. Anderson, E. Richardson, & N. A. Chambers (Eds.), *Cross-cultural caring: A handbook for psychologists* (pp. 59–94). Vancouver, BC: University of British Columbia Press.

Appendix E

Sikh Cultural Perspectives

1. Description of Cultural Spirituality and Health Themes

    a. A person's experience of life on Earth is influenced by karma (every action has a reaction). Humans can influence their destiny through their actions in life. Humans are reincarnated until eventually, under God's grace, they find their way to the feet of God and will be absorbed into the deity. Great emphasis is placed on purity: from proper foods to acceptable rituals, from community service to proper ceremonial celebrations, all help shape a future life. All of these cultural actions are mediated by the time-honoured traditions associated with Sikhism.

2. Conflicts and Distress

    a. Conflicts can be mediated by reference to scriptural teachings. There is a need to use traditional healing resources based on Sikh spiritual teachings because many Sikhs regard their scripture as the living embodiment of the Sikh Guru. The life-stress model has some potential in serving as a viable link between a Sikh holistic view of mental health and conventional counselling approaches. The life-stress model can best be described as an existential/spiritual approach holding that the human being wishes to fulfill four core human needs: security (*surakhia*), love (*prem*), respect (*izzat*), and freedom (*azzdi*) (*Guru Granth Sahib*, 1993, pp. 75–77). The four core needs in the life-stress model are interconnected and pursued simultaneously.

3. Social Supports/Family Caregiving/End-of-Life Preferences

    a. Sikh families often designate a spokesperson (usually the eldest son) to be responsible for managing issues of consent. Western society places a high value on individual autonomy in the decision-making process, whereas Sikhism stresses the importance of taking a holistic family/group approach to decision making. The client, his or her family, and the religion function as an integrated unit.

Review of Modules 1–4: Modesty Codes and Breast Cancer (LEARN Model)

Listen *respectfully to the client's perception of the problem. Get the cultural story.*

Listen to the underlying story of the elderly woman grappling with whether medical intervention is to be accepted or not. Note the various elements of the story that she gives prevalence to: the wedding of her grandson, her resistance to self-examination, and reluctance to make her health a matter of discussion at this critical moment, not to mention her resistance to discussing her problems with the eldest male in the family, her son.

Explain *your understanding of this family's cultural perceptions.*

Explain that you know that women of some cultures resist mammograms because of their invasive nature.

Acknowledge *the impact of cultural perspectives on traditional roles of family care.*

Acknowledge that the mammogram is a challenge for her values of modesty but that the tools for accurate determination are few. Acknowledge that technicians may not always be female, but that some steps might be taken to alleviate the potential for her encountering a male technician. Discover whether she will undertake self-examination as a potential basis for more accurately knowing the real reason for the pain. Acknowledge that kismet is a legitimate stance to take.

Recommend *a culturally sensitive health care solution.*

Recommend that she undergo meditations and prayers to determine what she should do, since the pain is not normal and it could indicate serious problems. Indicate a willingness to work with her, whatever her decision might be.

Negotiate *common ground that builds a competency bridge.*

Negotiate with a female family member close in age or with family ties to the elderly person to stress that the interventions you propose will not indicate anything more than diagnosis. Agree that larger issues will be left aside for future discussion.

Review of Modules 1–4: Helpful Hints for Culturally Sensitive Care Plan Solutions

1. **How have these modules made you aware of different cultural stories that relate to counselling care? Can you name some of the more important ones?**

Discussion points:

- Discuss the notion of "best care" when it acknowledges that cultural values are part of the equation.

- Discuss the role that religion plays in providing people a way of handling health risks.

2. **"Buy in" is a crucial element in counselling care. Can you describe why it is so important in ethnic contexts?**

Discussion points:

- Responsibility for one's health is often mediated by such things as family values, economics, and power structures between principals in the group. How does health care fit in these discussions?

- It is evident that elderly people take a different view of their health needs than younger members of the family. Discuss the way this feature plays a role in these modules.

3. **Why are end-of-life issues so prone to conflict within families?**

Discussion point:

- The agendas for families can often be very complex. Discuss some of the varieties in these modules.

4. **What role does differing interpretations of illness, wellness, and intervention play in defining health care? Is it possible to say that biomedicine is only one of several models?**

Discussion points:

- Despite more knowledge of health being available to ordinary people than ever before in human history, there is considerable lag between what people know and what they do about it. Are there examples in the stories presented in the modules of distinctive value leanings?

Review of Modules 1–4: Cultural Understanding (BRIDGES Tool)

Insight into the values, beliefs and attitudes of clients brings a deeper awareness of cultural perspectives. BRIDGES helps us gain deeper cultural understanding.

Beliefs, Values, Norms: In some cultures, there is an interplay of religious belief and health. The notions of kismet and karma are important in this film. Both mediate whether Marji will take steps to determine the source of her pain.

Roles and Relationships with Family/Relatives: The family—with its members occupying differing roles and having different expectations—is an important factor in health decision making. Leading males are accustomed to making critical decisions about family matters and must be consulted before major actions are undertaken. Yet the issue is complicated by this being an exclusively "women's" concern.

Identify Language, Literacy, Communication: The mother feels her role in and commitments to the family are more important than her own health. Sikhism tends to regard all issues in a holistic manner, and hence religious views are part of the discussion when it comes to health. No family member can emphasize one aspect of his or her life when it will impact the whole family.

Decision Making Methods/Practices: In order to have compliance in identifying and treating illness, it is important to consider the decision makers. It is important to involve the family to help the mother realize she is important and not just in terms of her role at the wedding. Marji would not make a health decision without bringing all dimensions of her life into the conversation, so she could not make an autonomous decision.

Group, Community, Organizations: In this Sikh family, support may be provided by the religious leaders and the community. Community life is organized around the temple or gundawara, where religious rites are performed and where religiously informed life takes place. Life's true course is held to be set within the rituals solemnized there.

Extraordinary Issues in Health (end-of-life, childbirth, etc.): These issues call for the commitment of the entire family, so Marji sees a conflict between the treatment of her own pain and the life-course event they are preparing for: the marriage of her grandson. Her own preference is to put her own problems behind the wedding plans.

Share Understanding of Cultures, Reach Common Ground, and Compromise: It is important to be aware of these norms, beliefs, and values, and develop common ground with the client and her family to reach a therapeutic treatment plan. Can Marji come to see the diagnostic test as an acceptable interim event before the wedding takes place? How is she to see its meaning within the family context? Some Sikh families may be more acculturated to Western values than is represented in this story, but the underlying value system can continue to play a role.

RESOURCE MATERIALS

Adamson, J. (2001). Awareness and understanding of dementia in African/Caribbean and South Asian families. *Health & Social Care in the Community, 9*(6), 391–396. http://dx.doi.org/10.1046/j.0966-0410.2001.00321.x

Ebrahim, S., Bance, S., & Bowman, K. (2011). Sikh perspectives towards death and end-of-life care. *Journal of Palliative Care, 27*(2), 170–174.

Guru Granth Sahib (Damdami Version). (1993). (G. Singh, Trans.). Amritsar, India: Sri Gurmat Press. (Original work published 1706).

Rao, A. S., Desphande, O. M., Jamoona, C., & Reid, C. M. (2008). Elderly Indo-Caribbean Hindus and end-of-life care: A community-based exploratory study. *Journal of the American Geriatrics Society, 56*(6), 1129–1133. http://dx.doi .org/10.1111/j.1532-5415.2008.01723.x

Lebrun, E., & Emblem, J. (2007). Spirituality and health in Punjabi Sikh. *Journal of Holistic Nursing, 25*(3), 141–148. http://dx.doi.org/10.1177/0898010106293592

Minhas, M. S. M. (1994). *The Sikh Canadians*. Edmonton, AB: Reidmore Books.

Puri, G. S. (1992). *Multicultural society and Sikh faith*. New Delhi, India: Falcon Faith.

Reimer-Kirkham, S. (2009). Lived religion: Implications for nursing ethics. *Nursing Ethics, 16*(4), 406–417. http://dx.doi .org/10.1177/0969733009104605

Sandhu, J. S. (2005). A Sikh perspective on life-stress: Implications for counselling. *Canadian Journal of Counselling, 39*(1), 40.

Appendix F

Hispanic Cultural Perspectives

1. Hispanic Protocols of Interaction

a. Many cultures resist the biomedical interpretations of psychological illnesses. They do this for several reasons that rest in cultural beliefs about illness, or because of social stigmas attached to someone prone to such illnesses. For many such cultures, mental problems are regarded as fatal flaws in the human character, and even something like dementia, which is clearly "physical" in origin, may be regarded as indicative of a personal flaw.

b. Many cultures also resist naming the lack of any kind in a personality as an "illness," purely because it empowers the person to skirt responsibilities by laying the blame on this personal "flaw." Naming it gives it authority to control someone's life.

c. Different cultures handle these issues differently. In this example, it is evident that the interpretation of Emilio's depression is mediated through his mother, who refuses to accept anything "mental" about her son. The result is a striking kind of dependence between mother and son that extends all the way to what is done with prescription medicine prescribed for Emilio by the physician.

d. There is a general reluctance in many cultures to treat mental health issues as illnesses, viewing them rather as evidences of faulty character or personal "weaknesses." Admitting to such a thing as mental illness can have important ramifications for social life: the people one can marry, the jobs one is allowed to do, and the roles taken in family power structures.

2. Hispanic Language and Communication

a. Reluctance to name Emilio's problem as mental leads to the construction of many story scenarios—from criticism of physicians who recommend psychological or psychiatric counselling to the use of herbals directed to certain kinds of personal weaknesses. Communications may avoid any reference to biomedical language, such as the word "mental," or even counselling as a way of denying the power of those words to turn a weakness into a medical problem.

b. Popular resistance to depression-as-illness indicates that the configurations of the mind are culturally defined. That is, many cultures do not accept the notion that the mind can be understood in a mechanistic way or that it is subject to scientific, causal understandings. The result is that people use language to build other meanings more compatible with their cultural viewpoint.

3. Provision of Health Care by Community and Organizations

   a. Many cultures assign psychological states to a range of experiences governed by religious and cultural institutions. That is, rather than assigning mental issues to medical care, home-spun remedies and even complicated meditation rites are used. Many stories are told of how these alternative therapies have been successful. Their popular success is often contrasted with medical procedures that are less effective. For some, it is the nature of the mind to be connected to emotions and matters "of the heart," so there is no clear reason why such matters need to be medicalized, since a church, religious groups, or a guru may provide successful therapies.

4. Decision Making and Caregiving

   a. In many cultures, caregiving is women's work, and some even accord curative powers to women, especially elderly women. The dominance of matriarchal authority is evident in Emilio's case, but there are many groups that value women as nurturers. This issue raises the further discussion of whether or not Emilio accepts responsibility for his own well-being.

5. Hispanic Beliefs, Values, and Health Care Outcome Expectations

   a. This story raises important issues about alternative therapies and the outcomes allegedly made by the physician's prescriptions in the face of a culture that does not accept the expectations built into pharmaceuticals. It also illustrates that mental health is subject to cultural viewpoints far more than other, more physical ailments.

6. Unique Mental Health Issues

   a. Diagnoses according to biomedicine may be accepted by some cultural groups, but obviously, when it comes to the mind, other perspectives can hold sway. The story illustrates the importance of "buy in" as an ingredient in counselling and psychiatric analyses.

Module 1: Resistance to Medical Interpretations of Depression and Mental Health (LEARN Model)

Listen *respectfully to the client's perception of the problem. Get the cultural story.*

Listen to Mrs. Gonzales's interpretation of her son's mental state, and note the emphasis she gives to the alternative viewpoint.

Explain *your understanding of this family's cultural perceptions.*

Explain that problems of the mind are very complicated and that several ways have been devised to deal with symptoms like Emilio has. Compare the approaches of the two physicians and place the differences into an alternative health care model in which the second may have had experience.

Acknowledge *the impact of cultural perspectives on traditional roles of family care.*

Acknowledge that we do not know all the causes of Emilio's problems but that there must be a way of making life easier for him. Acknowledge, too, that herbal medicine does assist some people and that believing in a solution can motivate people to get beyond how they feel at the moment.

Recommend *a culturally sensitive health care solution.*

Recommend that counselling professionals discuss together what medications Mrs. Gonzales uses, since Mrs. Gonzales regards it as important that the best herbals be used for her son's symptoms. Determine whether or not she will allow a procedure worked out with Emilio to work so that there may be some evidence on effectiveness.

Negotiate *common ground that builds a competency bridge.*

Negotiate with both the mother and the son, and insist on Emilio's commitment to whatever procedures you are able to negotiate with them. Indicate that you will work with whatever they agree upon so that you can build trust with them for future therapies.

Module 1: Helpful Hints for Culturally Sensitive Care Plan Solutions

1. **Several of these modules stress the ways in which differences impact health care. Can you enumerate some of the differences that cultural groups hold that differ from biomedicine?**

Discussion points:

- There are often significant differences between generations in terms of attitudes toward health issues. Discuss the importance of these for end-of-life care.

- Many cultures come to Canada with beliefs that are opposed to the way we practice medicine or treat health issues. Discuss how people's norms may change when they come to Canada, and point out how family decision making can change.

2. **Women play key roles in many of these modules, yet the role of informal caregiver is seldom recognized. What do these scenarios tell us about the informal caregiving situation?**

Discussion points:

- The history of medicine reflects how males have dominated conceptions of illness and therapy. Discuss how this bias may have skewed our perception of health care.

3. **Some people speak of complementary and alternative therapies as "witchcraft." How have these modules raised questions about that designation?**

Discussion points:

- Modern medicine is a fairly recent creation, yet it has resisted alliance with any "non-scientific" therapy. Discuss the issues related to this in the light of Emilio's story.

- Mental health issues and psychological treatments raise a storm of protest among many ethnic groups. Discuss why this is so.

Module 1: Cultural Understanding (BRIDGES Tool)

Insight into the values, beliefs and attitudes of clients brings a deeper awareness of cultural perspectives. BRIDGES helps us gain deeper cultural understanding.

Beliefs, Values, Norms: Understand that in some cultures, "mental illness" is a reflection of a personality or character flaw and may be stigmatized. This family identifies with its own norms, beliefs, values, and communication in regard to depression. The family holds that depression is not a medical illness but something that can be treated with psychosocial considerations and herbal remedies.

Roles and Relationships with Family/Relatives: In this culture, the mother has a strong role in caring for her son.

Identify Language, Literacy, Communication: The mother controls communications within the family and all communications regarding her son's condition go through her.

Decision Making Methods/Practices: In order to gain treatment compliance, it is important to consider the decision makers. In this situation, the mother is directing her son for treatment. Inclusion of the decision makers (here, the mother) is important for therapeutic treatment and management.

Group, Community, Organizations: In this family, support may be provided by the religious leaders and the community.

Extraordinary Issues in Health (end-of-life, childbirth, etc.): When people from other countries work in the Western world, there is a process of acculturation that may cause stress for clients and their families.

Share Understanding of Cultures, Reach Common Ground, and Compromise: It is important to be aware of these norms, beliefs, and values and to develop common ground with the client and his family to reach a therapeutic treatment plan that will help with this young man's healing process.

RESOURCE MATERIALS

Black, S. A., Markides, K. S., & Miller, T. Q. (1998). Correlates of depressive symptomatology among older community-dwelling Mexican Americans: The Hispanic EPESE. *Journals of Gerontology. Series B, Psychological Sciences and Social Sciences, 53B*(4), S198–S208. http://dx.doi.org/10.1093/geronb/53B.4.S198

Falcon, L. M., & Tucker, K. L. (2000). Prevalence and correlates of depressive symptoms among Hispanic elders in Massachusetts. *Journals of Gerontology. Series B, Psychological Sciences and Social Sciences, 55*(2), S108–S116. http://dx.doi.org/10.1093/geronb/55.2.S108

Gonzalez, H. M., Haan, M. N., & Hinton, L. (2001). Acculturation and the prevalence of depression in older Mexican Americans: Baseline results of the Sacramento area Latino study on aging. *Journal of the American Geriatrics Society, 49*(7), 948–953. http://dx.doi.org/10.1046/j.1532-5415.2001.49186.x

Krause, N., & Golden, L. M. (1991). Acculturation and psychological distress in three groups of elderly Hispanics. *Journal of Gerontology, 47*(6), S279–S288. http://dx.doi.org/10.1093/geronj/47.6.S279

Swenson, C. J., Baxter, J., Shetterly, S. M., Scarbro, S. L., & Hamman, R. F. (2000). Depressive symptoms in Hispanic and non-Hispanic white rural elderly: The San Luis Valley health and aging study. *American Journal of Epidemiology, 152*(11), 1048–1055. http://dx.doi.org/10.1093/aje/152.11.1048

Appendix G

Southeast Asian/Cambodian Cultural Perspectives

1. **Background on Southeast Asian Cultures**

   a. From 1975 to 1995, three million people left Vietnam, Laos, and Cambodia, including over 1.75 million Vietnamese. These peoples resettled in North America. The main reason for resettlement was the Vietnam War. Their own diversity, plus the differences between them, made the acculturation difficult. While many of these immigrants were Buddhist, a significant number were Catholic Christians.

2. **Health Risks in Southeast Asian Populations**

   a. A large number of refugees suffered from mental health concerns during the refugee experience, as well as a result of the sudden and involuntary cultural transplantation to a foreign culture, spending many years in squalid refugee camps, and being held in political detainee prisons in Vietnam for a decade or more (Mallica, McInnes, Pham, et al., 1998). In addition to the trials and tribulations of acculturation and adaptation to Western life, there were numerous stressors prior, during, and after refugee migration. The horrific life events experienced during the Vietnam War and its aftermath led to depression, loss, and trauma expressed as post-traumatic stress disorder (PTSD). The Southeast Asian elderly appear to be at higher risk of psychological distress than younger Southeast Asians because they have fewer buffer and coping strategies to deal with their distress (Shapiro, Douglas, de la Rocha, Radecki, Vu, and Dinh, 1999; Yee, 1997; Yee & Thu, 1987). Acculturation stress, depression, and mental health issues are not often incorporated into physical health research designed for Asian and Pacific Island (API) populations.

   b. Acculturation stressors, as measured by high cortisol levels, may be risk factors for cardiovascular and cerebrovascular disease, and cancer (Peeke & Chrousos, 1995; Schneiderman, Antoni, Saab, and Ironson, 2001). Opium and backache remedies containing opium continue to be used by Southeast Asian elders in North America to cope with acculturation stress (Smith & Nelson, 1991).

3. **Mental and Physical Health of Cambodians**

   a. Life expectancy in Cambodia is around forty-seven years for men and forty-nine years for women (Heng & Key, 1995). Many infectious diseases are the major cause of death in Cambodia (e.g., malaria, tuberculosis, severe anemia, under-nutrition, and diarrhea). In North America, chronic diseases are more commonly due to health compromised by acculturation.

b. The Cambodians are at high risk for post-traumatic stress disorder and depression, which are increased by financial stress (Blair, 2000). The majority of Cambodians in North American have been affected by genocide under the Khmer Rouge. Around two million Cambodians died in the Killing Fields from violence, starvation, and disease (Mollica, McInnes, Poole, and Tor, 1998).

c. One study found that obsessive thinking about loss of family members or traumatic events experienced in the Killing Fields was the root of the common illnesses among Cambodian elders. This condition (*pruit chiit/kiit chraen*) produces severe headaches with dizziness (Handelman & Yeo, 1996). Greater use of prescription drugs—for example, sleeping pills—is one result of coping.

d. Other studies have found that Cambodians present with functional vision loss or other symptoms due to conversion hysteria from traumatic wartime experiences. It is important to have a holistic medical approach when treating Cambodians who have suffered in the past, to recognize the symptoms of post-traumatic stress disorder (Drinnan & Marmar, 1991; Kinzie et al., 1998).

e. Cambodians have a high rate of chronic diseases (e.g., hypertension, diabetes, coronary artery disease, cerebrovascular accidents) as well as non-specific somatic complaints (headaches, dizziness, and fatigue) (Baughan, White-Baughan, Pickwell, Bartlame, and Wong, 1990).

4. Cambodian Health Beliefs and Traditional Practices

a. Khmer culture is a combination of Indigenous folk traditions and Indian and French influences (Zadrozny & Androsky, 1995). The majority of Cambodians adhere to Theravada Buddhism. The folk religion centres on spirits living in natural habitats—such as mountains—ancestral spirits, and dangerous spirits or ghosts. Some spirits are benevolent, while others are malevolent. Western medical practices were introduced to Cambodia around 1860; however, Indigenous practitioners were the first line of defence. Western physicians were seen only when the illness persisted. Indigenous practitioners dealt with sorcery and exorcised evil spirits from clients. Buddhist monks provided medical services ranging from spiritual to Western therapy. The causes of illness were typically attributed to supernatural causes or natural causes such as hormonal imbalances. Spirits cause illnesses by entering the body through the client's food. Practitioners of black magic can prevent or cause harm to people. Treatment may consist of ritual ceremonies to deal with the evil spirits, paying homage to the benevolent spirits, and use of herbal medicines.

5. Use of Medications

a. There is a belief that Western medicine is "stronger, faster, and curative," while folk medicine is "weaker, slower, but preventative." Such thinking has major implications for Southeast Asian elderly people's adherence to medical regimens. Decreasing drug doses is a cultural response to their perceptions about Western medication. Older Vietnamese and other Southeast Asian clients may decrease the prescribed dose and become non-compliant (Pham, Rosenthal, and Diamond, 1999). Some Cambodian clients may feel that the dose of medicine is too strong, due to their belief that Western medicines are powerful, and will choose to be non-compliant or decrease the dose (Shimada, Jackson, Goldstein, and Buchwald, 1995).

6. Southeast Asian End-of-Life Issues

a. Typically Southeast Asian elders prefer traditional values. Culture influences a variety of death and dying attitudes and medical decisions. Southeast Asian families have been influenced by religion and cultural philosophies, such as Buddhist beliefs about karma and reincarnation, with concerns for ancestral spirits. These beliefs may lead to an avoidance of hospitals, where lost souls—the souls of people who died did not have a place to rest—can gather and create havoc upon the living. Delayed medical attention may be the result of this avoidance of hospitals (Braun, Pietsch, and Blanchette, 2000).

b. Organ donation would be less likely in this population than in others because donors would be reborn incomplete, without all their vital organs, in the next life. Decisions to donate organs of dying elders by family members may be viewed as a sign of disrespect and as lacking in filial piety toward the family elder/ancestor (Nakasone, 2000). This behaviour may anger the family ancestor, who may create mischief for the living.

c. Heroic medical intervention, such as organ transplants or cardiac resuscitation with hospital strangers surrounding the dying client, may be regarded as disturbing the natural ebb of life and a sign of a "bad death" with accompanying negative emotions. At the same time, withdrawal of life supports may be viewed by Southwest Asians as causing or speeding the demise of their family elder. Palliative care, with its comforting, peaceful, and family supportive dimensions, may be more acceptable for Buddhists and other Southeast Asians. Many Vietnamese have been influenced by Catholic, Taoist, and Buddhist beliefs regarding life and death (Ta & Chung, 1990). There are cultural differences in death and dying truth-telling: some cultures do not speak of death; others regard it pragmatically (Crow, Matheson, and Steed, 2000; Muller & Desmond, 1992). Many Southeast Asian families do not want their physician to inform dying family members of their terminal prognosis because it would cause them to lose hope. There may be a belief that upsetting the loved one will bring death sooner, and this would show a lack of respect for the soon-to-be ancestor.

Module 5: LEARN Model Answer Key

Listen

Post-traumatic stress disorder occurs after experiencing or witnessing a highly traumatic event. Mr. Sylvan had a severe reaction to the Khmer Rouge's transfer of his family to a collectivist farm, known as the Killing Fields of Cambodia. He has intense recollections, flashbacks, nightmares, and distress when exposed to reminders of trauma, the triggers.

Explain

In Cambodia, Mr. Sylvan was taught that the best way to treat a traumatic event is to bury it deeply in his mind and never to revisit it. He feels that burying his feelings may help him avoid further nightmares and flashbacks. Yet Western counselling suggests that traumatic events should be talked about to remove the power they hold over a person's memory. The majority of Cambodians in North American have been affected by genocide under the Khmer Rouge.

Acknowledge

The Cambodian culture is a complex one, involving a combination of Indigenous folk traditions and Indian/Buddhist and French influences. The folk religion assumes that the natural environment is inhabited by spirits, some natural, such as mountain spirits; some ancestral; and some either benevolent or malevolent, such as ghosts. In Cambodia, there were Indigenous practitioners who dealt with sorcery and exorcised the evil spirits from clients, and Buddhist monks provided a range of therapies. Initial treatment may consist of ritual ceremonies to deal with the evil spirits or to pay homage to the benevolent spirits, or the use of herbal medicines. The basic belief was that only when these therapies proved unsuccessful might the client seek Western medical help.

Recommend

First, Dr. Brandon had to determine whether or not Mr. Sylvan believed his problem could be solved by traditional means. While Dr. Brandon did not ask him about spirit beliefs, he had to determine whether or not Mr. Sylvan believed his own therapies were satisfactory before he might commit himself to Dr. Brandon's therapy. If Dr. Brandon could not be sure of that, he could not really deal with Mr. Sylvan's problems. In some cases, he might have asked him how he felt about traditional methods, but in this case he recommended only that Mr. Sylvan commit himself to Dr. Brandon's help.

Negotiate

The common ground was the implicit understanding that Mr. Sylvan had come to: the realization that burying the trauma had not worked. He had to find a way to address the problems he was having, and Dr. Brandon's therapy at least offered a way around his trauma. Dr. Brandon built a competency bridge by offering him an alternative therapy to the one he had grown up with, and together they could adapt the therapy to Mr. Sylvan's current life.

Module 5: Cultural Competency Protocols Based on All Modules

In the film *Post-Traumatic Stress*, the client has suffered post-traumatic stress disorder as a result of his refugee experience. Use the film's story to determine some helpful hints for culturally sensitive care plan solutions that embrace the stories expressed in the modules.

1. **Cultures may have different ways of expressing the impact of mental stress, or have different ways of coping with illness. These have an impact on therapies offered by the health care professional. Looking over the several modules you have completed, can you indicate some of these perceptions?**

   Discussion points:

   - In key ways, relationships come into play when people are dealing with health issues. Often these relationships reveal cultural values arising from deep-seated beliefs. Discuss the ways these beliefs play a role in the cases you have reviewed here.

   - Many families have ways of relating to health care professionals that make it difficult to provide therapy. For example, some families closely guard information about health from the public and do not want to reveal it, even to professionals. Discuss how this feature of culture may have affected these cases.

2. **Responsibility for a family's well-being is often determined by gender. How does cultural difference regarding gender alter how therapy can be applied?**

   Discussion points:

   - The pressure of public shame has greater impact for some recent immigrant families than it does for some Western families. Discuss how this will influence the health care role you play.

3. **Have these modules helped you to see how your own culture may be nuanced differently?**

   Discussion points:

   - Mr. Sylvan's issue relates to a deeper issue. What is acceptable therapy for some kinds of illnesses?

   - Religious beliefs sometimes are the foundation for how a therapy will be accepted. Can you give some other examples of how this might be a challenge in a counselling clinic?

Module 5: Cultural Understanding (BRIDGES Tool)

Insight into the values, beliefs, and attitudes of clients brings a deeper awareness of cultural perspectives. BRIDGES helps us gain deeper cultural understanding.

Beliefs, **Values, Norms**: Many Cambodians adhere to Theravada Buddhism, a tradition that accepts many different kinds of spiritual realities in life as the believer seeks to eventually enter Nirvana. Moral values are also influenced by traditional beliefs in good and bad spirits present in the world that may impact a person's life. Generally, traumas are handled by "forgetting" them, suppressing them so that a person can carry on. Evil things happen in life and usually are associated with some bad influence, or perhaps even some bad action in a past existence. There may be some ambiguity about where the bad influence is coming from.

Roles and **Relationships with Family/Relatives**: The role of the family is a critical one for Cambodians, since family members contribute to one's well-being, and how one relates to them implies something about his or her karma. Cambodian moral thinking requires that one provide assistance to one's family first and foremost; to be available for family members is necessary for proper growth and proper spiritual achievement. Mr. Sylvan has to determine how much he was to "blame" for the destruction of his family, if at all. He has to confront the fact that he had apparently lost his ability to protect his wife and son, who are presumed deceased, so he needs to deal with his sense of loss both physically and spiritually.

Identify **Language, Literacy, Communication**: The transfer to Canada did not remove Mr. Sylvan from the problem of the destruction of his family. After spending many years in a refugee camp, he was transferred to Canada, whose values had little to do with his cultural upbringing. Canada did not provide him with a way to deal with his sense of loss. He felt alienated by language, demands, and his situation.

Decision **Making Methods/Practices**: This client would benefit from his spiritual leader to help bridge the culture to Canada, but he has to come to the point where he has to try a new and different therapy than he learned as a child.

Group, **Community, Organizations**: This client may benefit from support from a religious leader, such as a Buddhist monk or a sympathetic member of the Cambodian community.

Extraordinary **Issues in Health (end-of-life, childbirth, etc.)**: Trauma and war (refugee camps) are extraordinary situations that refugees often face. It is a major problem to understand why refugees have been made to suffer so much.

Share **Understanding of Cultures, Reach Common Ground, and Compromise**: It is important to be aware of these norms, beliefs, and values, and to develop common ground with the client to reach a therapeutic treatment plan based on his own coming to terms with his past.

RESOURCE MATERIALS

Baughan, D. M., White-Baughan, J., Pickwell, S., Bartlame, J., & Wong, S. (1990). Primary care needs of Cambodian refugees. *Journal of Family Practice, 30*, 565–568.

Blair, R. (2000). Risk factors associated with PTSD and major depression among Cambodian refugees in Utah. *Health & Social Work, 25*(1), 23–30. http://dx.doi.org/10.1093/hsw/25.1.23

Braun, K. L., Pietsch, J. H., & Blanchette, P. L. (2000). *Cultural issues in end of life decision making.* Thousands Oaks, CA: Sage.

Crow, K., Matheson, L., & Steed, A. (2000). Informed consent and truth-telling: Cultural directions for healthcare providers. *Journal of Nursing Administration, 30*(3), 148–152. http://dx.doi.org/10.1097/00005110-200003000-00007

Drinnan, M. J., & Marmar, M. F. (1991). Functional visual loss in Cambodian refugees: A study of cultural factors in ophthalmology. *European Journal of Ophthalmology, I*, 115–118.

Handelman, L., & Yeo, G. (1996). Using explanatory models to understand chronic symptoms of Cambodian refugees. *Family Medicine, 28*(41), 271–276.

Heng, M. B., & Key, P. J. (1995). Cambodian health in transition. *British Medical Journal, 311*(7002), 435–437. http://dx.doi.org/10.1136/bmj.311.7002.435

Kinzie, J. D., Denny, D., Riley, C., Boehnlein, J., McFarland, B., & Leung, P. (1998). A cross-cultural study of reactivation of posttraumatic stress disorder symptoms. *Journal of Nervous and Mental Disease, 186*(11), 670–676. http://dx.doi.org/10.1097/00005053-199811000-00002

Mollica, R. F., McInnes, K., Pham, T., Smith Fawzi, M. C., Murphy, E., & Lin, L. (1998). The dose-effect relationships between torture and psychiatric symptoms in Vietnamese ex-political detainees and a comparison group. *Journal of Nervous and Mental Disease, 186*(9), 543–553. http://dx.doi.org/10.1097/00005053-199809000-00005

Mollica, R. F., McInnes, K., Poole, C., & Tor, S. (1998, December). Dose-effect relationships of trauma to symptoms of depression and post-traumatic stress disorder among Cambodian survivors of mass violence. *British Journal of Psychiatry, 173*, 482–488. http://dx.doi.org/10.1192/bjp.173.6.482

Muller, R. F., & Desmond, B. (1992). Ethical dilemmas in a cross-cultural context: A Chinese example. *Western Journal of Medicine, 157*, 323–327.

Nakasone, R. Y. (2000). Buddhist issues in end-of-life decision making. In K. L. Braum, J. H. Pietsch, & P. L. Blanchette (Eds.), *Cultural issues in end-of-life decision making* (pp. 213–228). Thousand Oaks, CA: Sage Publications. http://dx.doi.org/10.4135/9781452204819.n14

Peeke, P. M., & Chrousos, G. P. (1995). Hypercortisolism and obesity. *Annals of the New York Academy of Sciences, 771*(1 Stress), 665–676. http://dx.doi.org/10.1111/j.1749-6632.1995.tb44719.x

Pham, T. M., Rosenthal, M. P., & Diamond, J. J. (1999). Hypertension, cardiovascular disease & health care dilemmas in the Philadelphia Vietnamese women. *Family Medicine, 31*(9), 647–651.

Schneiderman, N., Antoni, M. H., Saab, P. G., & Ironson, G. (2001). Health psychology: Psychosocial and biobehavioral aspects of chronic disease management. *Annual Review of Psychology, 52*(1), 555–580. http://dx.doi.org/10.1146/annurev.psych.52.1.555

Shapiro, J., Douglas, K., de la Rocha, O., Radecki, S., Vu, C., & Dinh, T. (1999). Generational differences in psychosocial adaptation and predictors of psychological distress in a population of recent Vietnamese immigrants. *Journal of Community Health, 24*(2), 95–113. http://dx.doi.org/10.1023/A:1018702323648

Shimada, J., Jackson, J. C., Goldstein, E., & Buchwald, D. (1995). Strong medicine: Cambodian views of medicine and medical compliance. *Journal of General Internal Medicine, 10*(7), 369–374. http://dx.doi.org/10.1007/BF02599832

Smith, R. M., & Nelson, L. A. (1991). Hmong folk remedies: Limited acetylation of opium by aspirin and acetaminophen. *Journal of Forensic Sciences, 36*, 280–287.

Ta, M., & Chung, C. (1990). Death and dying: A Vietnamese cultural perspective. In J. K. Parry (Ed.), *Social work practice with the terminally ill: A transcultural perspective* (pp. 191–204). Springfield, IL: Charles C. Thomas.

Yee, B. W. K. (1997). The social and cultural context of adaptive aging among Southeast Asian elders. In I. J. Sokolovsky (Ed.), *The cultural context of aging* (2nd ed., pp. 293–303). New York: Greenwood.

Yee, B. W. K., & Thu, N. D. (1987). Correlates of drug use and abuse among Indochinese refugees: Mental health implications. *Journal of Psychoactive Drugs, 19*(1), 77–83. http://dx.doi.org/10.1080/02791072.1987.10472382

Zadrozny, M. G. & Androsky, A. (Eds.). (1995). *Area handbook on Cambodia*. New Haven, CT: Juman Relations Area Files, Inc.

About the Authors

ROGER PARENT completed his PhD in semiotics and French-Canadian literature in 1992 at Laval University. Since then, he has taught mainly literature, theatre studies, and applied cultural semiotics at Campus Saint-Jean, University of Alberta. His research and publications deal with issues pertaining to theatre of creation, cultural development, and intercultural education. Based on his study of performance and culture, he has developed an interdisciplinary pedagogy and applied research methodology for resolving cultural conflict. His research and training methodology, along with accompanying learning materials, has been piloted nationally and internationally in collaboration with university and government partners in Canada, Europe, and Australia.

OLGA SZAFRAN is Associate Director (Research), Department of Family Medicine, University of Alberta. She obtained a masters in health services administration (MHSA) degree from the University of Alberta in 1985. Over the past twenty-eight years, she has been involved in family medicine research in the areas of health services, physician practice patterns, medical education, international medical graduates, and culture in medicine, and has published and presented in these areas. In the area of culture and medicine, Ms. Szafran co-edited *At the Interface of Culture and Medicine: Contemporary Studies* (2011), co-authored *Cultural Competency Skills for Health Care Professionals: Learning Manual* (2010), and co-produced eleven cultural teaching videos (2007, 2008, 2013).

JEAN TRISCOTT is professor and director of the Division of Care-of-the-Elderly, Department of Family Medicine. She graduated from medical school at the University of Alberta in 1981 and completed her residency in family medicine (CCFP) in 1983. Since that time, she has worked in the Northern Alberta Regional Geriatric Program (NARGP) at Edmonton General Hospital. She is a member of the Alberta Centre on Aging and the co-director of the Centre for the Study of Cross-Cultural Health and Healing. Dr. Triscott was involved in the development of the Memory Clinic in 1988, a service that provides early assessment of memory problems, as well as being linked to ongoing research programs in cognition and dementia, driving, participatory research in culture/end-of-life issues and dementia, geriatric, and chronic diseases.

EARLE WAUGH is professor emeritus of religious studies and director of the Centre for Health and Culture in Family Medicine at the University of Alberta. He currently heads up a research team on the intersection of culture and health. Together with Olga Szafran and Rod Crutcher, Dr. Waugh co-edited *At the Interface of Culture and Medicine:*

Contemporary Studies (2011). Dr. Waugh lectures and consults widely on health care and culture and has provided seminars for hospitals, pharmacy seniors, graduate physicians, and health care professionals throughout Alberta. He has received various awards for his work, including the 2010 Friend of Pharmacy of the Year award from the Alberta College of Pharmacists and the 2013 Sage Award for contribution to arts and culture in Edmonton.

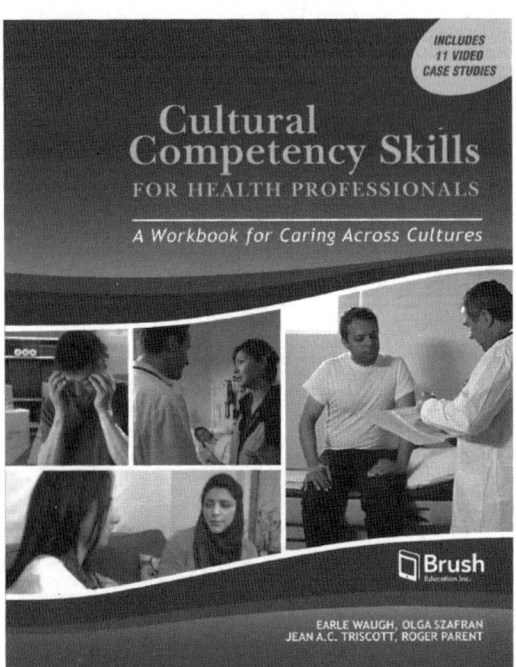